The Physician Scientist's Career Guide

Mark J. Eisenberg

The Physician Scientist's Career Guide

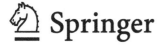 Springer

Mark J. Eisenberg
Divisions of Cardiology and Clinical
    Epidemiology
Sir Mortimer B. Davis Jewish General
    Hospital
McGill University
3755 Cote-Ste-Catherine Road
H3T 1E2 Montreal
Suite H-421
QC, Canada
mark.eisenberg@mcgill.ca

ISBN 978-1-60327-907-9   e-ISBN 978-1-60327-908-6
DOI 10.1007/978-1-60327-908-6
Springer New York Dordrecht Heidelberg London

Library of Congress Control Number: 2010934108

Printed on acid-free paper

Springer is part of Springer Science+Business Media (www.springer.com)

*Dedicated to Louise Pilote, my wife
and chief collaborator*

Strive not to be a success, but rather to be of value.

—Albert Einstein

Far and away the best prize that life offers is the chance to work hard at work worth doing.

—Theodore Roosevelt

Somewhere, something incredible is waiting to be known.

—Carl Sagan

Preface

The career of a physician-scientist is an exciting and rewarding journey. It is challenging, creative, intellectual, and requires perseverance and devotion. Being a physician-scientist means you have to balance two loves – clinical medicine and research. These loves are demanding but complementary – you will be a better clinician because you are a researcher, and you will be a better researcher because you are a clinician. As a physician-scientist, you have the unique privilege of being able to make meaningful contributions in the fields of patient care, teaching, and research.

In this book, I present some of the insider tips that I have learned over the past few decades as a physician-scientist. Most of these tips I learned through experience – very little was learned in a formal manner. Reading this book will expose you to some of the strategies, knowledge, and skills that will help your career flourish. For those just starting out on this path (medical students, residents, fellows, and junior faculty members), this book will help demystify the process of becoming and succeeding as a physician-scientist.

When reading this book, you may find it long on strategy, knowledge, and skills, but short on the love of science and discovery. In my experience, new physician-scientists do not lack motivation and ideals; what they lack is the practical ability to turn their ideas into grants and papers. This book tries to remedy that issue. Please forgive my lack of emphasis on science and discovery – I take that as a given. Traditionally, the knowledge and skills required to be a physician-scientist are learned by experience. The idea behind this book is that, with a few hours of reading at the beginning of your career, you will have a much better idea of what lies ahead. This book will not give you all the answers, but it will give you a map and compass to help navigate your own unique journey. The voyage that lies before you is one of the most rewarding and meaningful that you can imagine.

Montreal, QC, Canada   Mark J. Eisenberg

Acknowledgments

I wrote this book during a sabbatical year in Jerusalem, Israel. Just like most physician-scientists, my life is a frenetic balancing act – trying to maintain my research career, my clinical activities, and my family life. Without the leisure afforded by a sabbatical, I would not have been able to even contemplate writing this book.

My sabbatical year would not have been possible without the support of several institutions. I recognize that many universities in North America no longer award tenure and no longer support sabbaticals for physician-scientists. The fact that McGill still does is testament to its ongoing commitment to biomedical research. Without the protected time for research, the financial support, and the ability to take a sabbatical afforded to me by McGill, this book could not have come to fruition. Besides McGill, I am also indebted to the Hebrew University for awarding me a Lady Davis Sabbatical Fellowship and for allowing me to be a visiting professor at Hadassah Hospital. Finally, I would be remiss if I did not acknowledge the support of my cardiology group at the Sir Mortimer B. Davis Jewish General Hospital. My group provided encouragement, financial support, and coverage of my clinical responsibilities.

I am indebted to the Sir Mortimer B. Davis Jewish General Hospital, the Lady Davis Institute for Medical Research, and McGill for providing me with a safe haven in which I could develop my career as a physician-scientist over the past 15 years. In addition, I am indebted to the Fonds de la recherche en santé du Quebec, the Heart and Stroke Foundation of Canada, and the Canadian Institutes for Health Research. These three funding agencies have consistently provided me with the career awards and operating grants that I needed to succeed as a physician-scientist.

Importantly, I need to thank all my mentors, colleagues, trainees, graduate students, research team members, and patients over the course of many years. Much of what I have learned from them I have tried to put in this book.

Many individuals helped me with the practical aspects of putting this book together. Their activities included transcription, tracking down facts and references, and assembling tables and figures. I would like to extend my thanks to Mériam Abouelouafaa, Tara Baboushkin, Gabriel Cartman, Michael Coussa-Charley, Priyanka Dixit, Rebecca Fernando, and Brenda Matzov.

I particularly owe a very large measure of thanks to Heather Robinson who expertly coordinated this project over the course of many months and many drafts. She devoted an exceptional number of hours to this project. Without her, this book would not have been possible.

During my sabbatical year, I completed the International Masters in Health Leadership program in the School of Management at McGill. I discussed many of the management aspects of the physician-scientist pathway with both my classmates and my professors. I would like to thank them all for their insightful comments, and I would particularly like to thank Dr. David Colman, who supervised my final paper which included four chapters from this book.

My thanks also go out to several individuals who reviewed drafts of this book and offered many helpful suggestions. These individuals include Dr. Kris Filion, Robert Gorman, and Dr. Avi Shimony. In addition, I would like to thank the 16 anonymous individuals who agreed to be surveyed on issues related to improving the physician-scientist pathway.

Finally, I want to thank my family for supporting me in this project during our sabbatical year in Israel. Thanks go to my five children: Sarah Leah, Ariella, Elisheva, Elie, and Eliana. Most of all, I want to thank my wife, Dr. Louise Pilote, for insightful discussions about the physician-scientist pathway, for helpful comments that found their way into this book, and for reviewing the manuscript. Any success that I have had as a physician-scientist is due, in large part, to our successful collaboration over the two and a half decades since we first met as medical residents and discovered our mutual interests in medicine and research.

About the Author

Mark J. Eisenberg, MD, MPH, M. Mgmt is a tenured Professor of Medicine at McGill University and an associate member of the McGill Department of Epidemiology, Biostatistics and Occupational Health. He is a Staff Cardiologist at the Sir Mortimer B. Davis Jewish General Hospital in Montreal, Quebec, Canada and Director of Clinical Research of the McGill Cardiology Fellowship Program. In addition to his clinical responsibilities as an interventional cardiologist, he is Director for the Cardiovascular Health Services Research Group and a Principal Investigator at the Center for Clinical Epidemiology and Community Studies at the Jewish General Hospital.

Dr. Eisenberg completed an AB (cum laude) in Chemistry in 1980 at Cornell University in Ithaca, NY and then an MD at the University of Rochester School of Medicine and Dentistry in 1985. Following his MD, he did a residency in Internal Medicine at the Royal Victoria Hospital, McGill University, and obtained a Masters of Public Health degree at Harvard University. He completed a research fellowship in Echocardiography and Epidemiology in 1992 at the Cardiovascular Research Institute of the University of California at San Francisco followed by a clinical cardiology fellowship at the University of California at San Francisco in 1994. In 1995, after finishing a fellowship in interventional cardiology at the Cleveland Clinic, Dr. Eisenberg took up a post as an assistant professor at McGill University. He became an associate professor in 2002, received tenure in 2005, and became a full professor in 2008. In 2010, Dr. Eisenberg completed a Masters degree in Management at McGill University.

Dr. Eisenberg has published over 160 peer-reviewed articles in journals such as the Annals of Internal Medicine, Circulation, the Journal of the American Medical Association, Lancet, and the New England Journal of Medicine. He has been first or senior author on close to 100 of these publications and has received funding for over 50 grants. He is a fellow of both the American College of Cardiology (ACC) and the American Heart Association (AHA) and has served as a member of the Task Force on Clinical Expert Consensus Documents for the ACC since 2004. He has been an internal and external reviewer for multiple peer-reviewed funding agencies. He instructs medical students, residents, and fellows at McGill University and teaches Continuing Medical Education courses. As a research supervisor, he has mentored close to 100 undergraduate, medical, and graduate students, as well as large numbers of residents and fellows. His research interests include clinical trials, cost-effectiveness studies, health services and outcomes research, meta-analyses, primary and secondary prevention of cardiovascular disease, systematic reviews, and smoking cessation.

Dr. Eisenberg is married to Dr. Louise Pilote, an academic internist and health services researcher. They have five children.

Contents

Part I
Getting Started as a Physician-Scientist

To be successful, the first thing to do is fall in love with your work.

–Mary Lauretta

Chapter 1
Beginnings

Try a thing you haven't done three times. Once, to get over the fear of doing it. Twice, to learn how to do it. And a third time, to figure out whether you like it or not.

–Virgil Garnett Thomson

Introduction

Before offering my tips for building a successful career as a physician-scientist, let me first tell you how my career came about. If you want to get right to the details of the knowledge and skills needed to be a physician-scientist, go right to Chapter 2. However, if you are not sure if this is the right career path for you, read about how I became a physician-scientist. If my story resonates with you, this may be the right career for you as well. Every physician-scientist has a unique story about how they arrived at where they are. Here is mine.

Early Years

When I was growing up in Rochester, New York, my father was a gastroenterologist/internist and my mother was a nurse, so medicine was in the atmosphere at our house. Neither of my parents was involved in research, but discussion of clinical activities was the norm. By late high school, I knew I wanted to be a doctor. I briefly considered being an English major during my undergraduate studies at Cornell University, but I knew I wanted to go to medical school, so I needed to fulfill the prerequisites. I took a number of English courses and enjoyed writing, but I chose to major in chemistry and spent several years doing research in a biochemistry laboratory. I found the work to be intellectually appealing, but it did not "grab" me, and I was not particularly successful at it. Although my mentor and other people in the lab were supportive, I never published any papers, and I found the work to be repetitive and distant from any practical applications. In retrospect, I was searching for a research outlet but found bench work unfulfilling. At the time, I was completely unaware of the existence of clinical research.

M.J. Eisenberg, *The Physician Scientist's Career Guide*,
DOI 10.1007/978-1-60327-908-6_1, © Springer Science+Business Media, LLC 2011

During my college years, I had several other experiences that affected my future career. I spent one summer working in a hotel in Switzerland, another in a biochemistry research laboratory within a large pharmaceutical factory in a small town in France, and another "shadowing" several physicians at a local hospital, including my father, a general surgeon, and a radiation oncologist. My experiences in Europe opened me up to different cultures and different ways of doing things. I found that I was interested in languages and people. My summer in the hospital confirmed my desire to be a doctor.

Medical School

The first inkling that I might be interested in becoming a physician-scientist came during the required introductory epidemiology course in medical school at the University of Rochester. The majority of my classmates found this course to be dry and remote from direct patient care. It was one more course to get through before getting on with the "real" work of being a doctor. I, however, loved it. It was the first time that I was really enamored by a particular field of medicine. Because of the course, I decided to apply for a scholarship to do a summer research project. Once accepted, I chose to work with my father on identifying risk factors for gastritis. I wanted to examine potential determinants like alcohol consumption, aspirin use, and smoking. I was also interested in psychological determinants, such as individual anxiety levels versus the impact of major life events like the death of a spouse or the loss of a job. Neither my father nor I had any training in clinical research. Nevertheless, I tried to correlate risk factors that I documented in a patient survey with the biopsy results of patients who underwent gastroscopy. I presented my results as a poster at Medical Student Research Day. After Research Day, my mother put up the poster in our basement, where it remained for close to two decades. Whenever I returned home, I looked at that poster and I could see the first awakenings to my future career. I could see that even then, I had a deep-seated urge to do clinical research even though I did not have a clear idea of what it was and had not yet met any clinical researchers. That summer research project was my first foray into the world of clinical research.

While discovering the world of clinical research, I was still interested in languages and cultures. I decided to take a year off between my second and third years of medical school and go to Israel. In Israel, I spent six months at an intense Hebrew language school in a development town in the Negev desert. The following six months I spent in Jerusalem doing bench work in one of the hospitals. We were trying to establish a relationship between low magnesium levels following myocardial infarction and an increased incidence of cardiac arrhythmias and sudden death. I found the experience to be unfulfilling. The project itself was interesting. However, my job was to separate lymphocytes from blood and help analyze them for magnesium levels. I had little patient contact and no involvement in data analysis or writing; activities that I had really enjoyed during my summer project on gastritis.

My research experience in Israel confirmed that I was not cut out for a career in bench research. Nevertheless, my interest in cardiology was kindled.

After my return from Israel, I had a difficult time re-adapting to medical school. There was little outlet for my creative energies, and I felt cut off from my experience with other languages and cultures. However, I had a transformative experience during my fourth year of medical school. I spent a month doing a cardiology elective with a well-respected cardiologist who was both a clinician and researcher. Over the course of the month, I got a good look at this man and his career. Several aspects of the way he handled his career were attractive to me. First, he was a model clinician. He spent time with his patients and was truly empathetic, in addition to being very rooted in the science of cardiology. Second, he had an eclectic professional life. He rounded on his patients in the hospital, had an active clinic, and ran large multi-center clinical trials. I recall two episodes in particular that greatly influenced me. One morning, we made rounds in the hospital. I saw him step out of the elevator with an unshaven face and an unkempt appearance. It turned out that he had been up all night with a sick patient. I thought to myself, "Here's a doctor that I would like to emulate." Second, in the doctor's private office, we saw a patient who was complaining of fatigue. The patient was bradycardic with a heart rate in the 20s and an ECG showing complete heart block. The doctor personally drove him to the emergency department. This was the type of behavior that I could respect and relate to.

This clinician asked me to write a paper over the course of my month's elective with him. This was an unusual request; clinicians never ask medical students to write papers during clinical electives. Nevertheless, I jumped at the task. I wrote a review article about magnesium deficiency and cardiac arrhythmias. I felt that although I had been involved in this area during my research time in Israel, I never had the chance to explore the science and the theory behind it. I enjoyed researching and writing the paper, and my mentor encouraged me to submit the paper for publication. It was one of the biggest thrills of my life when it was accepted and published. The experience of researching, writing, and publishing a paper was very fulfilling, and it encouraged me to explore clinical research during my residency in internal medicine.

Residency

After completing medical school, I went to the Royal Victoria Hospital, McGill University, Montreal, Quebec to do a residency in internal medicine. My first ward rotation confirmed my interest in cardiology. My clinical rotations also raised many questions that I wanted to explore in closer detail. When I came up with a clinical question while seeing patients, I reviewed the literature and often found that there were no definitive answers to my questions. Thus, I felt that there was a potential career for me as a physician-scientist, in which I could explore practical questions that came up when seeing patients.

One of the questions that I developed early in my internship was the following: what is the value of blood-work obtained during in-hospital cardiac arrests? I was frequently called in the middle of the night when a patient had a cardiac arrest. I would perform CPR, defibrillate the patient, place a central line, and administer vasopressors and anti-arrhythmic agents. During these arrests, we routinely drew blood and sent it emergently to the laboratory to be analyzed for electrolytes. We were looking to see if hyperkalemia was the cause of the patient's cardiac arrest. The laboratory results often came back when the patient was already declared dead. Not unusually, hyperkalemia was present. I felt that hyperkalemia was the result of the dying process rather than the initiator of an arrhythmia which caused the arrest. I wanted to explore this issue in more detail.

To that end, I approached one of the staff cardiologists about doing a research elective with him. I told him about my project, and he told me about another project he wanted me to work on. I spent a month working on both projects. For my project, I went to the biochemistry laboratory and asked them to write down the name, date, and time for every patient who had stat electrolytes drawn during a cardiac arrest. I also asked them to add calcium and magnesium to these requests. By the end of the year, I had a list of one hundred patients who had experienced an in-hospital cardiac arrest and had electrolytes drawn during the arrest. I then did a chart review and documented the electrolytes that were drawn prior to, during, and after the arrest – if the patient lived. However, when I brought the results to my supervisor, he could not really help me analyze them. He did not have the expertise or statistical background for these kinds of analyses. This was also true for the study he had me involved in. In the end, I had a large collection of data but no way of analyzing it.

At the time, there were few physicians with epidemiology backgrounds. There was only one in our hospital, and it was difficult to gain access to him. Personal computers and user-friendly statistical software were not yet in common use. To do preliminary analyses on the results, I had to go to the Department of Epidemiology and Biostatistics to type all the data into a mainframe computer. The types of analyses I was able to perform without any outside help were not adequate to write up either of the projects that I had started. Despite this obstacle, I was very taken with the idea of doing clinical research. I liked the idea of being able to focus on a single research question and bring it to some sort of resolution. I presented my preliminary data at Resident's Research Day and won an award for it.

By the time I was a second-year resident, I knew that I wanted to become a physician-scientist. I needed to investigate the different ways to train for a career in this area. I found out about the one-year Master of Public Health degree program at the Harvard School of Public Health. The program was two years for most applicants, but for applicants who were already physicians, the program could be done in one year. I applied and was accepted for entrance between my second and third years of residency. Although this program broke up my residency, I really wanted to discover whether this was a career path I wanted to pursue. I felt that I needed to dedicate some time to this question.

Harvard School of Public Health

My year at the Harvard School of Public Health was probably the most fruitful academic year of my entire career. I was excited by every course that I took. I took a variety of courses, including biomedical writing, biostatistics, environmental science, epidemiology, and healthcare management in the developing world. About half of my classmates were from overseas, representing many different countries. Many of these individuals were older, with experiences in the developing world. I learned a lot from my classmates.

I had to write three major papers over the course of the year, and I tried to write them in such a way that I could publish them as review articles. I wrote one paper on leprosy in the developing world, in which I recounted my experiences during a one-month dermatology elective in India during my residency. I wrote another article looking at the geographic variations of magnesium levels in drinking water and their relationship with the incidence of sudden death. I also wrote a paper on the incidence and prevalence of rheumatic fever and rheumatic heart disease in the developing world. Each of these papers was written for a course and was subsequently published.

Perhaps most importantly, I brought the data from my residency research projects to one of the emeritus professors as part of an independent tutorial course. Once a week, this professor suggested a new way to analyze the data. I then used my newly developed computer skills to perform the analyses. Each week, I would return with my analyses, and he would suggest some other way to analyze the data. By the end of the semester, I had fully analyzed the data and written two research articles that were subsequently published.

In addition to finishing my research articles, I gained some insight into the real world of epidemiology from this professor. He had been the head of the data and safety monitoring board for the Physicians' Health Study. This was a large clinical trial in which physicians were randomized to receive aspirin or placebo. Based on the results of this study, many individuals began taking daily aspirin to prevent nonfatal myocardial infarctions. The manner in which the data were presented in the article was not entirely to the liking of my mentor. The primary endpoint of the trial was all-cause mortality. During an interim analysis, the data and safety monitoring board found that there was no difference in all-cause mortality between individuals receiving aspirin and those not receiving aspirin. For this reason, they recommended stopping the trial early because of futility (i.e., no likelihood of finding a mortality difference even if the trial was continued). However, the published results emphasized the secondary endpoint of nonfatal myocardial infarction and seemed to suggest that this was the primary finding of the trial. The investigators reported that there was a significant reduction in nonfatal myocardial infarction with aspirin use. They minimized the fact that overall mortality was no different between the two arms of the trial. The run-in period with this trial was also not widely discussed after the trial was published. During the run-in period, all patients received aspirin, and only those who did not have GI distress and who could tolerate aspirin were actually randomized. Thus, this trial, which is the basis for the widespread use of aspirin for primary prevention in North America today, had several problematic issues that were not widely discussed in the medical literature. My experiences with this emeritus professor were very positive and gave me a sense of the inside world of epidemiology and clinical trials.

Transition

At the end of my year at the Harvard School of Public Health, I returned to Montreal for my final year of internal medicine residency. During that year, I interviewed for cardiology fellowships. The program that I was most impressed with was at the University of California, San Francisco (UCSF). At the time, the program was a four-year fellowship as opposed to a three-year program everywhere else in the US and a two-year program in Canada. Nevertheless, I decided to rank this program first. The program involved two years of research followed by two years of clinical cardiology. I was fortunate enough to be accepted. In addition, I organized it in such a way that I was able to take another year off between my residency and my cardiology fellowship.

Back to Israel

Between my residency and my cardiology fellowship, I went back to Israel. In Israel, I performed research under the guidance of a physician involved in a large international multicenter trial. I did a sub-study analysis while I was with him. Unfortunately, I had limited access to my supervisor. Although this was not my most fulfilling learning experience, I did produce two papers. One paper was the sub-study work that I had to do mostly by myself. The second came about because of a friendship that I developed with one of the residents at the hospital. Together we wrote up and published a case report about the association between cytomegalovirus infection and thrombocytopenia.

Cardiology and Research Training

In July 1990, I began my cardiology fellowship at UCSF. Because my first two years of fellowship were pure research, I decided that I wanted to develop a clinical skill at the same time. I could not do research in any of the invasive areas, because I had not yet done any clinical cardiology training. For that reason, I chose to do two years of echocardiography/research.

I worked in an echocardiography laboratory headed by Dr. Nelson Schiller. Nelson is an internationally known echocardiographer and one of the fathers of quantitative echocardiography. Prior to his involvement, echocardiography had largely been a subjective imaging technique. Nelson helped to bring quantitative measures into echocardiography; variables like ventricular wall thickness and chamber diameters were directly measured. Standards were developed, and subsequent guidelines were based on his work. During my time in his laboratory, I really blossomed as a researcher. I had limited night and weekend call and my clinical responsibilities of performing and reading echocardiograms were light. Thus, I had time to spend on research.

During those two years, I initiated a total of 15 papers, all of which were ultimately published. These papers were a mix of case reports, case series, cohort studies, and experimental studies. I found that I really enjoyed the process of collecting and analyzing data and writing papers. This clinical research experience was highly motivating for me. I was in a world-class center surrounded by physician-scientists who were really fascinated by research. I developed collaborations with other physicians at UCSF. I did several studies with a psychiatrist who was examining the effects of cocaine. I did studies where I performed transthoracic and transesophageal echocardiograms while subjects were receiving intravenous cocaine, to see its effects on the coronaries and left ventricular function. I also did an echocardiographic sub-study of a very large cohort study on perioperative ischemia. This paper was published in the *Journal of the American Medical Association*. Thus, I had a very fruitful research experience as a cardiology fellow at UCSF. There were opportunities available for me to present abstracts at large international meetings, and I also had the opportunity to attend a 10-day epidemiology seminar sponsored by the World Heart Federation in Rio de Janeiro. Each of these experiences helped solidify my decision to become a physician-scientist.

Following my two years of research, I completed two years of clinical cardiology. When I finished my clinical cardiology training at UCSF in 1994, I decided to do a year of interventional cardiology at the Cleveland Clinic. This turned out to be a pivotal year in my career. The research milieu at the Cleveland Clinic was very different from the ones I had previously experienced. At that time at McGill, clinical research was more of an individual craft that was practiced by rare individuals in relative isolation. At UCSF, research was more organized but still not a large-scale endeavor. At the Cleveland Clinic, clinical research had been perfected into an organized, large-scale process. Dr. Eric Topol, a world-renowned researcher and principal investigator of the GUSTO trials, was the chair of the department of cardiology. There were close to 50 cardiology fellows at the Cleveland Clinic, including eight in interventional cardiology. Virtually everyone submitted abstracts to the American College of Cardiology meetings and the American Heart Association meetings each year. Eric had a close collaboration with Dr. Rob Califf who ran the data coordinating center at Duke. I recall that Eric came around during the summer to each of the interventional fellows with a long list of topics and instructed us to pick out five topics each and to draw up empty tables for the data that we needed. He then had the empty tables faxed to Duke. These tables were subsequently sent back with the data filled in, and then we wrote the abstracts. This was my first experience with secondary data analysis from large clinical trials.

During my year at the Cleveland Clinic, I became an interventional cardiologist and performed many angioplasty procedures. However, I also wrote a number of papers as first author and as a collaborating author. I noted one problem with this training process though. Several of the cardiology fellows I was training with also wrote papers during their year in Cleveland. However, these individuals often did not have organized research experiences such as I had at the Harvard School of Public Health and UCSF. The fellows wrote articles which were published in moderate to high-impact journals, but they did not really have much methodological background or the experience of collecting and analyzing data themselves. They were presented with the data and then wrote the papers. Thus, when they went on to establish their own careers, they had little experience in conducting their own research projects. Although it was understood that they had received research training as part of their interventional fellowship, they did not, in fact, have the full scope of training necessary to become successful physician-scientists.

At the Cleveland Clinic, I also observed that in order to become a maximally productive physician-scientist, you need to leverage your abilities by forming a research team. You can produce only one or two papers per year if you are the only one designing the projects, collecting the data, analyzing the data, and writing the papers. With a team, however, many of the mundane tasks can be delegated and the principal investigator can focus on coming up with ideas and overseeing the conduct of the research. When you have a well-managed research team, you can produce a large number of high-impact publications. I was very impressed with the research process at the Cleveland Clinic, and I sought to emulate this on a smaller scale when I came back to McGill.

Principal Investigator

I returned to McGill University as a new assistant professor in July of 1995. Because I was not Canadian, I was unable to obtain a medical license immediately. At the time, I was very frustrated. I felt that my angioplasty skills were getting rusty. It was six months before I was able to begin doing clinical activities again and work in the cardiac catheterization laboratory. However, this setback turned out to be a blessing in disguise. During those six months, I was able to sit in my office writing grants and finishing papers. This opportunity gave my career a jumpstart, which was at least partially responsible for my subsequent success.

My father once told me that you learn the most during your first year in practice. This proved to be true for me, particularly in terms of becoming a physician-scientist. In July, I was expected to begin writing grant proposals for submission in September. I had never even seen a grant proposal before, let alone written one. I spent the entire summer writing a grant proposal for a large clinical trial with a budget of well over $1 million. I submitted the grant proposal to the Heart and Stroke Foundation of Canada. I then found out that the maximum they fund in Quebec is $25,000 per year for three years. This was a major strategic error on my part. I was clearly responsible for not having sought out a mentor or sufficiently researched the guidelines of the funding agency. McGill did not have a program in place for new investigators to have formal mentors. There was no process for new investigators to have their grants reviewed before they were submitted. I found that, although I was an accomplished investigator for my stage, I had insufficient experience at identifying good research ideas for grant proposals and no experience actually writing grant proposals.

My first few years at McGill were a struggle to develop the knowledge and skills I needed to succeed as a physician-scientist. Virtually everything I learned was by trial and error. I often wished that I had a career guide that spelled out all the things I needed to know. Now that I am mid-career and on sabbatical with time to reflect and write, I have put together all my "trade secrets" in this book. I hope you find them useful.

Summary

Every physician-scientist has a unique story to tell. There is no right or wrong pathway to becoming a physician-scientist. In order to succeed, you need to acquire the knowledge and skills that can be obtained only by training in a variety of laboratories with a variety of mentors. Focused research training is a must. In this book, I have tried to present many of the lessons I have learned during my own odyssey as a physician-scientist. I hope that recounting the lessons I learned will help you navigate the physician-scientist pathway.

Key Points

- There are many different pathways to becoming a physician-scientist.
- Try research early on in your training to see if you want to pursue it.
- Spend focused time on research to help decide if this is the career for you.
- Find physician-scientist mentors to see if this career appeals to you.
- Try different types of research, different labs, and different mentors to discover what appeals to you the most.

Chapter 2
Is a Physician-Scientist Career Right for You?

> *The first step to getting the things you want out of life is this: decide what you want.*
>
> –Ben Stein

Introduction

Early in your training, you will need to consider whether a physician-scientist career is right for you. To help you make this decision, this chapter examines the following questions: what is a physician-scientist? What types of research do physician-scientists conduct? How do you determine if you are suited for a career as a physician-scientist? And how do you become a physician-scientist? If you have already embarked on the physician-scientist pathway, I still encourage you to read this chapter. An important part of being a physician-scientist is to nurture the next generation. We train students in our laboratories, provide career advice to trainees, and serve as role models for the next generation. For these reasons, we need to articulate what a physician-scientist is, what we do, why it is important, and how aspiring physician-scientists can get started.

What Is a Physician-Scientist?

A physician-scientist is a practicing clinician who spends the bulk of his or her time doing research (Table 2.1). They usually work at academic medical centers. Like other academic physicians, physician-scientists are involved in teaching, administration, and clinical activities. However, physician-scientists are especially dedicated to generating new medical knowledge. Their role is important, because they identify novel and clinically relevant questions at the bedside and have the knowledge and tools to study these questions in the laboratory. They take their laboratory results and apply them back at the bedside.

M.J. Eisenberg, *The Physician Scientist's Career Guide*,
DOI 10.1007/978-1-60327-908-6_2, © Springer Science+Business Media, LLC 2011

Table 2.1 Physician-scientists versus clinician-educators

	Physician-scientists	Clinician-educators
Career	Spend the majority of their time in research and less in clinical work	Spend part of their time in clinical practice and part in teaching
Description	Investigate clinical questions that arise in practice to improve understanding and develop better treatments and practices	Implement new knowledge into practice and share it with students
Focus	Disease-oriented basic science research Application of basic science findings to patients Dissemination of research results Clinical investigation of patients Population and public health research Health services and systems research	Patient care Educational, evidence-based practice, dissemination methodologies
Place of practice Education	Academic medical centers Clinical training Additional research training Usually a Master's or a PhD Two–three years post-doctoral research fellowship	Academic medical centers Clinical training Possibly a Master's May include specialization in educational theory/practice

1. Branch WT, Kroenke K, Levinson W. The clinician-educator – present and future roles. J Gen Intern Med 1997; 12(Suppl 2): S1–S4.
2. The Clinician Scientist: Yesterday, Today and Tomorrow. http://www.cihr-irsc.gc.ca/e/12970.html. Accessed April 7, 2009.

What Types of Biomedical Research Do Physician-Scientists Perform?

Biomedical research can be loosely divided into four subsets: (1) basic science research; (2) translational research; (3) clinical research; and (4) population research (Table 2.2). Physician-scientists balance their clinical activities with one or more of these areas of research. For example, I work as an interventional cardiologist. I spend 50% of my time on clinical activities like performing angiograms, angioplasties, and stress tests, rounding in the CCU, rounding on the cardiology consult service, as well as working one half-day in clinic every other week. I spend the other 50% of my time doing clinical and population research related to cardiology.

Basic Science Research

Basic science research is focused on developing a better understanding of both normal and abnormal functioning of the human body. It does not usually have a

Table 2.2 Types of research

Type	Description
Basic science	• Increases knowledge and understanding of underlying disease processes • Does not involve human subjects • Examines molecular and cellular mechanisms of pathogenesis • Conducted in the laboratory
Translational	• Translates scientific discoveries into practical, human applications • Requires mastery of basic sciences, technology, and laboratory techniques
Knowledge translation	• Ensures that new treatments and research knowledge reach intended patients or populations and are implemented correctly • Implements strategies for improving the use of or adherence to treatment • Requires mastery of clinical epidemiology, evidence synthesis, communication theory, public policy, & mixed methods/qualitative research
Clinical	• Applies basic science and translational research in patients • Tests new knowledge, treatments, devices, etc. in patients • Direct application to patient care • May lead back to the laboratory to refine treatments for human usage • Observational or interventional
Population	• Studies human subjects to improve the health of populations • Identifies population-based risk factors and interventions to prevent onset of, interrupt the progression of, or improve population-based disease

1. Questions about Clinical Research. http://www.niehs.nih.gov/research/clinical/join/questions/index.cfm#clinical. Accessed March 25, 2009.
2. NIH Roadmap for Medical Research: Translational Research. http://nihroadmap.nih.gov/clinicalresearch/overview-translational.asp. Accessed May 19, 2009.
3. What is clinical research and what are human clinical trials? http://www.ncabr.org/biomed/FAQ_general/faq_gen_5.html. Accessed March 27, 2009.
4. Stevens LM. JAMA patient page. Basic science research. JAMA 2002; 287: 1754.
5. Taylor HA, Johnson S. Ethics of population-based research. J Law Med Ethics 2007; 35: 295–299.
6. Thomas C. Between bench and bedside – which research manuscripts are truly translational? Gastroenterology 2009; 136: 1484–1486.
7. Woolf SH. The meaning of translational research and why it matters. JAMA 2008; 299: 211–213.
8. Zucker DR. What is needed to promote translational research and how do we get it? J Investig Med 2009; 57: 468–470.

direct application to patients, but it provides the foundation that ultimately leads to improved understanding of the disease process and improved methodologies to prevent or modify it. Basic science research usually involves laboratory work far removed from patients. It can involve disciplines such as medical genetics and molecular biology.

Translational Research

Translational research spans the gap between basic science findings and actual clinical applications. It takes novel findings from the basic science laboratory and applies them directly to the patient. Translational researchers use tools common to the basic science researcher, but they also conduct research involving patients. Recently, the term translational research has been subdivided into two types: T1 and T2. T1 translational research involves taking basic science findings and developing them into practical applications such as vaccines, pharmaceuticals, and diagnostic tests. T2 translational research is also known as knowledge translation research. This type of research disseminates results to pertinent stakeholders and seeks to translate results into practice.

Clinical Research

Clinical research involves human subjects but encompasses different types of study designs. Cross-sectional studies examine a group of patients who have a particular clinical syndrome or disease. Case-control studies compare patients with a particular outcome to patients without that outcome. Cohort studies follow patients with a particular exposure to an agent or event or belonging to a particular group and examine their clinical outcomes. Clinical trials randomize patients to one experimental treatment or versus placebo. Clinical research can also involve meta-analyses, where published studies are pooled together statistically to provide more robust estimates of the efficacy of a new treatment. Systematic reviews, where all the medical literature on a particular topic is reviewed in a systematic way so that conclusions can be drawn to influence practice, are also a type of clinical research.

Population Research

Population research is focused on improving the health of individuals and populations by studying questions that can only be answered by examining large numbers of patients. Population research often involves the use of large administrative databases to examine questions that cannot be investigated with smaller data sets. It also includes disease surveillance and population-level interventions. The results of these investigations are frequently used to guide healthcare policy at the institutional or government level. For example, the association between a recently released medication and a rare adverse event might be identified only in a large administrative database study.

Research and Clinical Activities

In addition to research, physician-scientists are involved in patient care, teaching, and administrative responsibilities. Individual physician-scientists vary widely with respect to how much of their time is available for research activities. Some physician-scientists spend almost all their time conducting research, while others spend 50% or less on research. Most individuals who spend less than 50% of their time on research do not fit the classical definition of a physician-scientist. However, some senior physician-scientists have progressively taken on so many administrative activities that less than 50% of their time is devoted to research. If they are still productive researchers, I still consider them to be physician-scientists.

At the beginning of your career, it is often difficult to know how to apportion your time. Some physician-scientists who spend most of their time on research would be happier with greater exposure to patients. Conversely, some of those who spend much of their time on patient care would prefer to have more time for research. It is essential to establish a solid research program early in your career. For this reason, reserve the majority of your time for research. If you wish to spend more time on patient care once your research program is firmly established, you can easily move in that direction after a few years. It is difficult to move in the opposite direction. If only 20% of your time is protected for research early in your career, it will be difficult for you to establish a strong research program; without a strong research program, it will be difficult to convince your supervisor to provide you with additional protected time. Consequently, strive to devote 80% or more of your time to research when you begin your career as a physician-scientist. This percentage can easily be reduced later if you so desire.

What Is a Clinician-Educator?

Most physicians who practice in academic medical centers are not physician-scientists. In many institutions, these academic physicians are called clinician-educators (Table 2.1). The term clinician-educator indicates that the individual is both an excellent clinician and teacher. Clinician-educators spend most of their time seeing patients, teaching medical students, residents, and fellows, and performing administrative activities. The clinician-educator track has been developed at many academic medical centers to recognize the accomplishments and services provided by non-physician-scientists. At these centers, a separate set of promotional criteria have been established for clinician-educators. The traditional promotion track was skewed in favor of physician-scientists, and the chance of being promoted without substantial research accomplishments was limited. In the clinician-educator track, non-physician-scientists have a greater opportunity to advance academically based on their teaching, research, and administrative accomplishments.

At most academic medical centers, there is a large amount of clinical work to be done. If every academic physician were a physician-scientist, there would not be enough physicians to perform the clinical work. As a result, in most centers, the majority of physicians are clinician-educators. Clinician-educators do the bulk of the patient care, thereby protecting the time physician-scientists can devote to research. Although it is reasonable for an academic department head to expect that all members of his or her department be actively involved in some form of research, it is understood that the majority of the members of any department spend most of their time performing clinical activities.

Qualities and Skills Necessary to be a Physician-Scientist

You need to identify the type of career that will bring you the most satisfaction and allow you to make your greatest contribution to patients and society at large. If you think that a career as a physician-scientist will fulfill these needs, then determine at an early stage in your training whether you have the qualities necessary to be successful as a physician-scientist. You need to be intelligent, motivated, hard-working, and efficient. You also need to be a self-starter, an excellent problem solver, and an effective manager. You should enjoy being challenged by difficult problems, have a high tolerance for frustration and failure, be able to balance multiple projects at once, and be dedicated to and interested in the discovery and creation of new knowledge.

A physician-scientist requires an eclectic skill set. It is possible to be a successful physician-scientist even if you are weak in one or two of the skills required. However, if you lack skills in several domains, it is unlikely that you will be successful. For example, you need to be skilled at and enjoy biomedical writing. If you are not a good writer, it is possible to improve this particular skill. However, if you do not believe yourself capable of writing papers and grant protocols for the rest of your life, the physician-scientist career is probably not for you. Other skills you need to develop during your training are the following: the ability to identify compelling and fundable research questions; the perseverance to work on projects for months and years at a time; the ability to manage a research team; and the ability to collect and analyze data. If you cannot or do not want to develop these skills during your training, you might want to consider another career path.

Are You Suited for a Career as a Physician-Scientist?

Most physician-scientists identify their interest in research early in their medical careers, and many identify this interest while they are still medical students. Some begin by completing a combined MD–PhD degree program. Others get their first research experience during a medical school summer break or during a year off from medical school. Some perform their first research projects as residents or fellows. It is important to identify your interest in research as early as possible. The best way to identify whether you are suited for a career as a physician-scientist is to conduct a research project. Once exposed to the process of identifying a research problem, collecting and analyzing data, and writing a manuscript, you will be able to determine whether you enjoy the experience and whether you want to be involved in these activities as a significant part of your career. Only then can you move on to deciding how to obtain the necessary training.

Paths to a Physician-Scientist Career

Different people identify their interest in combining research and clinical practice at different stages of their training. There are multiple combinations of clinical and research training that can prepare you for this career, but different training programs are more appropriate depending on when you identify your research interest.

Early Bloomers

Some students identify an interest in research prior to entering medical school. These students are often referred to as "early bloomers." Their interest is frequently kindled during a research experience prior to or while attending university. For those who identify their commitment to research early on but who want to spend some time doing clinical work as well, the MD–PhD program is an excellent option.

MD–PhD Degree

The MD–PhD degree, a medical scientist training program established in both the United States and Canada, is excellent preparation for a career as a physician-scientist. Many universities in North America allow medical students to obtain a PhD during the course of their medical training (see Appendices 1 and 2 for a list of training programs). Typically, you go through the first two years of basic science training with the rest of the medical school class. Then, while the rest of your class goes on to the third and fourth years of medical school, you complete your PhD. The PhD requires three or more years. Once you have completed the PhD requirements, you return to do the third and fourth years of medical school.

MD–PhD programs were established to increase the number of physician-scientists. Most graduates go on to become physician-scientists, with the majority performing basic science or translational research. Very few graduates perform clinical or population research. The MD–PhD program has several benefits. First, if you are accepted into an MD–PhD program, your tuition to medical school is usually waived. Because of the high cost of medical school, this is a very attractive alternative. Second, the MD and PhD degrees are often completed in less time than it would take to complete an MD and PhD separately. Credit is often given toward the PhD for courses taken during the basic science years of the MD degree. Finally, the combination of the MD–PhD degree may allow you to integrate your clinical and research experiences in a way that sequential degrees would not.

The MD–PhD degree has several disadvantages, however. First, there is a significant time lapse between the second and third years of medical school while you work on your PhD. It can be difficult to re-enter the clinical world as a third-year medical student after such a long break. This can be difficult from a social perspective as well, since your cohort from the first two years of medical school has moved on without you. Second, your research area during your PhD may not correspond with your final career choice. It is often not until the third and fourth years of medical school, or even residency, that you identify which clinical area is of most interest to you. You may obtain a PhD in neuroscience, for example, but find after clinical exposure that you prefer obstetrics. Although some of the techniques obtained during your PhD may be useful in any field, it might be helpful to delay your research training until you identify your particular area of clinical interest, so that you can get relevant specialized training in that area. Finally, after obtaining a PhD, most individuals complete the third and fourth years of medical school, residency, and subspecialty training. By the time you are an assistant professor ready to begin your research career, much time has passed since your laboratory training. By that time, your laboratory skills may be rusty, and it may be difficult for you to compete with pure PhDs who just completed their training. Consequently, many graduates of the MD–PhD program go on to do additional post-doctoral training before starting their first job.

Late Bloomers

Physician-scientists who do not obtain their research training in MD–PhD programs are sometimes referred to as "late bloomers." Late bloomers are individuals who identify their research interests during medical school, residency, or subspecialty training. As opposed to individuals in the MD–PhD programs, late bloomers typically obtain their specialized research training sometime after medical school.

For an aspiring physician-scientist, it is preferable to become involved in research as soon as possible. This often means during medical school. Over the course of four years of medical school, a student can be exposed to research projects with several different supervisors. While medical schools provide an overview of the entire field of medicine, exposure to a particular research supervisor and one or more research projects can provide in-depth understanding of a particular field. Early research experiences are often the catalysts that help you develop a career as a physician-scientist. To facilitate this, most medical schools offer scholarships to students to conduct research during summer or winter breaks or part-time during the school year. Research supervisors often have ideas for multiple research projects but lack the time to complete them all. Medical students can provide the legwork required to advance many research projects, while discovering whether or not this career path appeals to them. With the help of a keen medical student, many successful research projects have been accomplished.

Some medical schools allow students to take a year off to do research. For example, I took a year off and went to Israel where I conducted research on magnesium deficiency and cardiac arrhythmias. As a result of this project, I ultimately became a cardiologist and a physician-scientist. My career start was not atypical. Many medical students have worked with me during their training. Many of them published articles in high-impact journals and developed a sophisticated understanding of a particular area that they never would have achieved without the focus of a research project. Most importantly, conducting a research project while a medical student provides you with significant insights into whether being a physician-scientist is an attractive career goal for you. At the beginning of medical school, most students have only a vague idea of what a physician-scientist is. During the course of their training, however, they come into contact with many physician-scientists. Although medical students may decide to follow such a career path, they often do not know how to develop a similar type of career. Working closely with a physician-scientist helps them discover how to proceed along this career pathway.

If you have not performed research as a medical student, I encourage you to get involved as either a resident or a subspecialty fellow. During both residency and subspecialty training, there are elective periods when you will have the opportunity to be involved in research. These periods are excellent times to identify whether a physician-scientist career is a viable option for you. The more research projects you are involved in, the easier it will be to decide whether this career will suit you.

Very Late Bloomers

Very late bloomers are individuals who become physician-scientists late in their careers. Although unusual, very late bloomers do occur and are sometimes quite successful. These physician-scientists are often full-time clinicians or clinician-educators who practice medicine for many years and then decide to make a contribution to research. Virtually all of them take time off from their careers to go back to school to obtain an additional degree, such as an MSc in Epidemiology, an MPH, or even a PhD. I know a number of clinicians who followed this career path. Several of them have become extremely successful. The late bloomer pathway, although feasible, requires a lot of time, effort, and determination.

Additional Research Training

Virtually all physician-scientists obtain focused research training in addition to their clinical training. It is unusual to see a successful physician-scientist who has not spent at least one year doing focused research training. The more time you spend obtaining and honing the necessary research skills, the more likely you are to be successful. One mistake I frequently see among aspiring physician-scientists involves their choice of additional research/clinical training programs following their subspecialty training. They spend one or two years at another center obtaining a particular clinical skill. During that time, they write several papers. When they begin their first jobs as new assistant professors, they begin on the physician-scientist career track. However, several years later, their research careers flounder, because they have trouble obtaining grants and publishing papers. The reason for their failure is often that their research training did not, in fact, focus on how to become an independent researcher. Many clinical/research training programs offer opportunities to be involved in different facets of the research process, without teaching all of the skills involved or providing an opportunity to see a project through from start to finish.

Research training needs to provide you with the skills required to identify a viable, fundable research project, to design studies, to write solid grant proposals, to collect and analyze data, to write manuscripts, to correspond with journals, and to publish papers. You also need to learn how to review manuscripts, review grants, and manage a research team. Many individuals who complete additional training after their fellowships are overly focused on learning a particular clinical skill. They may have the experience of writing an original research article based on data from a previously established database or the experience of writing a review article that is published in a high-impact journal. However, these experiences are not the same as obtaining focused research training that provides you with the skills you need to become a successful and independent physician-scientist.

Choosing Your Training

Decide whether you want to complete a formal research training degree program or an informal supervised experience with someone who is established in the field. In my opinion, it is better to obtain formal training. A Master's or PhD degree adds credibility to your research credentials and will help you obtain a position as a junior faculty member. When selecting an institution or a mentor, ensure that the experience can provide training in the specific skills your future career will require. In addition, consider the reputation of the program and the mentor within the academic community.

Master's Degrees

Many physician-scientists obtain an additional degree during their research training. If you are not prepared to spend the time necessary to obtain a PhD degree, there are several Master's degree programs that will give you the bare essentials needed for a career as a physician-scientist. Many physician-scientists who obtain Master's degrees go on to perform clinical or population research, while most physician-scientists who conduct basic science or translational research obtain PhDs. Perhaps the most common Master's degrees are the Master's of Public Health (MPH) and the Master's of Science in Epidemiology. There are also one-year programs with very specific foci, such as training in clinical trials or cost-effectiveness. These programs can be valuable to an aspiring physician-scientist.

MPH degrees can be obtained at many universities in North America and overseas, including Berkeley, Harvard, Johns Hopkins, North Carolina, Yale, and the London School of Hygiene and Tropical Medicine. Some MPH degrees are general in scope, like the one I completed at the Harvard School of Public Health. Others are focused on topics like epidemiology, biostatistics, or maternal and child health. At McGill, the MSc in Epidemiology degree has traditionally been a two-year program. The program can be thesis- or non-thesis-based. An MSc in Epidemiology gives you a solid base in the principles needed to perform clinical research.

Other Master's degrees can provide you with focused training in a particular discipline, but these degrees are not traditional routes for a career as a physician-scientist. These degrees include an MSc in Education, a Master's of Public Policy, a Master's in Quality Assurance, and a Master's in Health Care Management. Although these degrees are not traditionally research-oriented, they do provide focused training in areas that are pertinent to medicine and that could potentially be used as a focus for a career as a physician-scientist.

PhD Degrees

Some physician-scientists complete a PhD after finishing their clinical training. My wife, for example, did a residency in internal medicine, followed by a Robert Wood Johnson fellowship in clinical epidemiology, and then a PhD in Epidemiology at Berkeley. She then returned to McGill, where she works as a physician-scientist combining cardiovascular health services research with a career as an academic internist.

When obtaining a PhD following your clinical training, the amount of time you dedicate to finishing the degree may be less than that required if it is completed prior to your MD degree. Typically, you need to be on campus only for course work. If you are organized and efficient, the research and thesis can be completed while you are working as an academic physician. This career track is an option if you want to become a basic scientist with only a small amount of your time dedicated to clinical practice. Whereas obtaining a PhD as part of an MD–PhD program involves years of clinical training during residency and fellowship before you return to the laboratory, obtaining a PhD after your clinical training allows you to hit the ground running. When you begin work as a new assistant professor, you are in command of the latest laboratory techniques. Whether you complete a PhD following your clinical training or as part of an MD–PhD program, you may ultimately need to do a post-doctoral fellowship to be competitive with pure PhD biomedical scientists.

Timeline for Training Programs

Most individuals obtain their focused research training after residency. You should examine potential training programs at least one year before you wish to begin your training, and you should explore training awards at least nine months before. However, each institution and funding agency has its own timelines, so the earlier you look into them, the better will be your chances. More detailed information about choosing and applying for a training program is presented in the next chapter.

After Training

Your career as a physician-scientist really begins when you start your first job and receive an appointment as an assistant professor. Most new assistant professors obtain similar agreements when they start their careers as physician-scientists. Your time is usually protected for research for a period of three–five years. During that period, you need to obtain an operating grant and generate solid publications. In some institutions, you will need to obtain a career award as well. At the end of this period, if you are unsuccessful, you will likely be obliged to switch to the clinician-educator track. Therefore, if you want to be a physician-scientist, it is important to get a good start. Develop the skills required before you become an assistant professor. You need to have excellent clinical training as a medical student, resident, and subspecialty fellow. In addition, you will require at least one and preferably many years of additional research training. The more years of focused research training you obtain, the more likely you will be to succeed. Although there are many career trajectories that will enable you to become a successful physician-scientist, they all follow the same common pathway: obtaining a combination of excellent clinical and excellent research training.

Summary

Whether you are contemplating a career as a physician-scientist or are already a physician-scientist and are mentoring trainees, it is important to have a clear picture of what this career entails and how to move it forward. Every physician-scientist has a unique story about how they arrived at where they are. There are no right or wrong paths. The key is to obtain excellent clinical and research training and to have the desire to include medical research as an important component of your career.

Key Points

- A physician-scientist is a practicing clinician who spends substantial time doing biomedical research.
- Physician-scientists are also involved in patient care, administration, and teaching.
- A clinician-educator is a practicing clinician and teacher who does not spend substantial time doing research.
- There are four main areas of biomedical research: basic science, translational, clinical, and population-based.
- Most physician-scientists spend $\geq 50\%$ of their time on research.
- Get started in research as soon as possible by participating in projects during medical school, residency, and fellowship.
- Obtain as much focused research training as possible.
- Learn to identify fundable research questions, write research proposals and articles, collect and analyze data, and manage multiple projects at the same time.
- New assistant professors typically receive three–five years of protected time for research, during which they need to obtain an operating grant, generate publications, and optimally obtain a career award.

Suggested Reading

1. Andriole DA, Whelan AJ, Jeffe DB. Characteristics and career intentions of the emerging MD/PhD workforce. JAMA 2008; 300: 1165–1173.
2. MD-PhD Dual Degree Training. http://www.aamc.org/students/considering/research/MDPhD/start.htm. Accessed March 27, 2009.
3. Brand RA, Hannafin JA. The environment of the successful clinician-scientist. Clin Orthop Relat Res 2006; 449: 67–71.
4. Hare GM. Challenges and rewards of the clinician scientist career path. Clin Invest Med 2008; 31: E302–E303.
5. Haspel RL, Orlinick JR. Physician-scientist training. JAMA 2006; 295: 623–624.
6. Marban E, Braunwald E. Training the clinician investigator. Circ Res 2008; 103: 771–772.
7. Rosner B, Nayak J. The Complete Guide to the MD/PhD Degree. 1st ed. Alexandria, VA: J & S Publishing Company; 2004.
8. Rosser W. Bringing important research evidence into practice: Canadian developments. Fam Pract 2008; 25(Suppl 1): i38–i43.
9. Taylor RB. Academic Medicine. 1st ed. New York, NY: Springer Science+Business Media; 2006.
10. Teo AR. The development of clinical research training: past history and current trends in the United States. Acad Med 2009; 84: 433–438.
11. Whitcomb ME. The need to restructure MD-PhD training. Acad Med 2007; 82: 623–624.

Chapter 3
Training as a Physician-Scientist

The path to success is to take massive, determined action.
                                                              –Tony Robbins

Introduction

You have decided to investigate whether being a physician-scientist is the right career for you. At this point, you should have some experience doing a variety of research projects, but you have little formal research training. To become a successful physician-scientist, you will need to pursue focused research training. Focused research training often comes between the end of your clinical training and your first job as a physician-scientist. These years are critical, because it is during this time that you develop the skills needed to succeed as a physician-scientist. Focused research training requires at least one and often many years to be dedicated to research. It often involves obtaining an additional degree such as a Master's or a PhD. It may also involve working in a laboratory in another city for extensive training and development of laboratory skills. In this chapter, I discuss the following topics: choosing a research training program; applying to training programs; choosing a primary and several secondary research topics; and what to avoid during research training.

Choosing a Research Training Program

Most physician-scientists are late bloomers who decide to obtain focused research training after their clinical training. They become interested in research in medical school, residency, or fellowship. They may have done a research elective with an individual who sparked their interest, or they might have spent a summer or winter break doing research. In some way, they developed an interest in research and are considering it as a career option. However, they do not yet have the tools to succeed as physician-scientists. To acquire these skills, they will need at least one and more likely several years of additional research training.

M.J. Eisenberg, *The Physician Scientist's Career Guide*,
DOI 10.1007/978-1-60327-908-6_3, © Springer Science+Business Media, LLC 2011

There are several ways to identify potential research training programs. The best way is to speak to mentors and other senior investigators who are already established in the field you are interested in. You can also do a quick Medline search for individuals who are actively publishing in your area of interest. Once you have developed a list of possible programs and training directors, contact them to see if they accept trainees or can recommend someone who does.

Stay or Go?

One of the first considerations when choosing a research training program is whether you should stay at your current institution or go to another one. If possible, I highly recommend that you go to another institution. You may have excellent training facilities at your institution, but you probably have done years of clinical work and several research projects there. It is important to see how research is conducted in other laboratories and institutions. Sometimes, there are family responsibilities or other issues that preclude you from leaving your city. This is understandable, but I encourage you to relocate for one or more years of focused research training if feasible. If you cannot relocate to a new city, go to a different laboratory or institution in your own city or perhaps commute to a nearby area. Exposure to a different institution allows you to become a more well-rounded physician-scientist and provides you with the opportunity to develop new collaborators and mentors, thereby making you a more attractive candidate when you apply for your first position.

Other Considerations

When you are looking for a research-training program, many considerations need to be taken into account. If you are married, you need to consider what your spouse will do. If you have children, you need a place where there are good schools. Obviously, the primary issue is to determine where you will get the best research training. To find where you can obtain the best research training, you will need to consult with many individuals. Discuss the issue with mentors at your current institution. Once you have developed a list of potential research training programs, you can obtain more detailed information.

Begin by reading journal articles that have come out of the laboratories you are interested in. Is the laboratory director always the first author or do the trainees get to be first authors on the manuscripts? What is the productivity of this laboratory? Are their articles published in important journals? Examine their departmental and institutional websites. Specific training programs and laboratories often have their own websites. These websites typically include a list of research interests, selected publications, the CVs of investigators, and a list of past trainees. Looking at the website of a laboratory can help you decide whether it is the right place for you. It is also worthwhile to contact people who have already gone through that laboratory.

For example, if you are interested in going to a particular program in a particular city, contact that laboratory and speak to a couple of the individuals working there. What are they learning? Do they think it is a good experience? Do they think that the laboratory director is a good research mentor? What has happened to other individuals who trained in this laboratory? How many years did they need to obtain research training there? You can also contact individuals who trained in the laboratory and who are now physician-scientists and solicit their opinions.

Funding

Another important consideration is how to fund your research training. In some cases, if you are applying as a full-time research trainee, your laboratory director will have funds available. In other cases, you may be responsible for applying for your own training grant. Funding agencies in the United States, Canada, and other countries have various types of awards available. These awards are not intended to support clinical training; they are intended to support focused research training. Training awards are intended for individuals who will spend 80% or more of their time on research. They may be conducting clinical work in conjunction with their research, but research is the main focus of their activities.

The deadline to submit applications for training awards is often nine months or more before your start date. Applications require you to have a designated supervisor and a specific project. It is helpful to start researching funding possibilities early on. It may be worthwhile to apply for these awards even if your supervisor is able to fund you. This demonstrates your ability to obtain competitive, peer-reviewed awards, as well as potentially providing you with supplementary funding for your work.

Tips for Applying to Training Programs

Once you develop a list of potential training programs, create a personal statement and CV. Your personal statement is generally a one-page letter describing who you are, what your training is, and what kind of research training you want to obtain. It should not be a "Dear Sir or Madam" letter; rather, it should be written directly to the director of the training program or laboratory you are interested in. Be honest in this letter. Tell them exactly how much research training you have, what you hope to learn in their laboratory, and what assets you will bring to the laboratory. In one paragraph, describe your research training to date. If you have high-impact publications, mention them in this paragraph. Be clear about what you are looking for. Indicate how many years you want to spend at their institution. If possible, include specific information about the laboratory you are applying to. This information can be gleaned from your mentors or from a review of the laboratory's website. Your CV should accompany the cover letter. The next chapter will describe the elements of an academic CV.

Laboratory directors have a lot of experience in looking at cover letters and CVs. They can quickly see whether you are intelligent, thorough, and enthusiastic; whether you have been productive; and whether you are likely to be productive in the future. In addition, they are experienced biomedical writers. If you have errors in grammar and punctuation in your cover letter and CV, it will be obvious to them. Such errors, as well as inconsistencies in formatting and presentation, will reduce their interest in having you in their laboratory. After preparing a draft of your cover letter and CV, ask your mentors for their comments before sending it out.

Reference Letters

In addition to sending a cover letter and a CV, it is useful to have reference letters sent separately. Individuals with whom you have done research projects at the medical student, residency, or fellowship level typically write these letters. If you are already a practicing physician, ask your colleagues for reference letters. Carefully consider whom you ask for reference letters. Be frank when discussing whether they can write a strong letter for you. Asking something like, "Do you think you know me well enough to write a strong letter?" gives them the opportunity to gracefully decline if they do not feel they can recommend you. If you do not think that they can give you a positive letter, do not ask them. It is better to have one or two strong letters than to have five unenthusiastic letters.

Phone Calls

In addition to having your mentor send a letter to the program director, it is very helpful if they can make a phone call on your behalf. The best-case scenario is applying to a training program where your mentor trained. In that case, your mentor may have a close relationship with the director and can recommend you as a major asset to the laboratory in a more personal way. A direct telephone call can be a strong calling card. It is much stronger than a reference letter. Slots at training programs are often highly contested. Be as competitive as possible. This means that you need to have a strong cover letter, a strong CV, strong reference letters, and if possible, a phone call extolling your virtues to the laboratory director.

Track Record

Perhaps your most important asset is your track record. If you have never participated in a research project and have never written a paper, it is unlikely that a laboratory director is going to be enthusiastic about taking you on. The stronger you make your publication record prior to applying for a training program the better. The best predictor of future productivity is past productivity.

Several institutions offered me a position based on my track record in research. For example, when I applied to the Cleveland Clinic for an interventional cardiology/research fellowship, I was one of many individuals applying for eight slots. Thirty other aspiring trainees interviewed on the same day as I did. We were all dressed similarly, and we all had similar clinical backgrounds. Ultimately, I was accepted for one of the positions. I believe I was chosen because I already had an MPH from Harvard as well as an extensive publication track record for my stage. The following year, when I applied for a position as a cardiologist and physician-scientist at McGill, my research training and publications set me apart from other applicants in terms of what I could offer to the hospital and the university.

When training institutions and laboratory directors look at potential trainees, they are looking to see whether an individual is a good fit for their laboratory. Not only do they want someone who is personable, enthusiastic, and who will work well as a member of the team, but they also want someone who is going to be productive. It is much more attractive for them to have a trainee who is a self-starter, who has ideas for research projects, and already has experience doing research. First author publications are one of the best ways of demonstrating this to a prospective research supervisor. They show that you have experience following a project through. You generated an idea, collected data, and wrote most or all of a paper. First author publications demonstrate that you have actual experience being a productive researcher. Your strongest attribute when applying for a research-training program is your prior track record in research. Keep this in mind as you are doing your clinical training. Get as much research experience as you can prior to applying for a formal research training position.

Interviewing

I will cover the topic of interviewing in detail in the next chapter when I discuss getting your first job. However, after you send your cover letter, CV, and reference letters (hopefully followed by a telephone call from one of your research mentors), you will likely be invited to an interview. This may occur in the context of a meeting with the prospective laboratory director at a medical conference or may involve a trip to the laboratory itself. In either case, be prepared. It is helpful to have mock interviews beforehand. Arrange these with your mentors. Anticipate the questions that will be asked and prepare your answers in advance. You also need to come to your interviews with questions of your own – questions like the following: what have previous trainees done after they left your laboratory? What is the typical profile of the trainees that come to your laboratory? What projects do you have going on currently? What projects do you think I would be involved in? What techniques, skills, and knowledge will I learn in your laboratory? What is the duration of training? What kinds of seminars and workshops go on in your laboratory and in your division? What is the typical productivity of a trainee in your laboratory? Do trainees typically get to be the first author on papers? Will there be a salary or grants supplied (and if so, for what amount?) or do I have to obtain support on my own? All of these questions should be addressed in your interview.

First impressions are important. Dress well and be punctual. Demonstrate that you are a team player and that you have the requisite traits and experience to be an asset to the laboratory. Interviews for research training programs are very important. They give you a good idea of what goes on in the laboratory and whether it will be a good fit for you. Carefully evaluate whether the projects will be interesting for you in the long term. The interview gives the laboratory supervisor an idea of whether you are appropriate for their laboratory. During the interview, carefully evaluate whether the laboratory supervisor will be a good mentor for you. Are they a physician-scientist? Will you be able to relate to them? Do they have command of the tools and skills and knowledge that you want to obtain? You may want to develop basic science laboratory skills and are considering a laboratory with a pure PhD laboratory supervisor. If so, will this experience give you enough clinical exposure? Will you be able to relate to this individual? These are the types of questions you need to ask yourself. Once you complete your interviews, discuss the results with your mentors and with your spouse to decide which is the best training program for you.

Choosing Research Projects

Once you arrive at your research training program, you will need to develop a primary research project to work on. I highly encourage you to develop several secondary projects as well. These secondary projects should involve only a small amount of your time, but will allow you to have multiple publications by the time you complete your training. The focus should be on your primary topic. Give substantial thought to what your primary project will be. In most cases, your laboratory supervisor will have several potential topics for you to work on. During your initial interview, you will likely have considered some of these topics. Now is the time to decide what you are going to work on.

Primary Research Project

There are several considerations when deciding what your primary research project will be. Is it feasible? How much time will be required to finish the project? How many publications can you reasonably expect the project to generate? Will these publications appear in high-profile or low-profile journals? When you apply for your first job, will this research project be viewed as compelling? Most importantly, will work on this project give you the skills and knowledge you will need to be a successful physician-scientist. For example, if you are an internist pursuing a PhD in epidemiology, there are many areas of epidemiology that you could pursue. You could focus on clinical trials, the secondary analysis of large administrative databases, the performance of large cohort studies, the methodology of meta-analyses, pharmacoepidemiology, and so on. You need to be sure that the training you choose will provide the right skills.

Whatever it is, your primary research project will provide you with skills and knowledge about a particular area. It is very likely that this will be your primary field of interest for many years once you begin your career as a physician-scientist; as a result, carefully consider your choices. If you do not see yourself doing secondary analysis of large administrative databases for a decade or more, do not choose a topic in this area as your primary research project. If you are interested in clinical trials, get specialized training in this area. Seriously consider what area of research you want to focus on. Once you make your choice, search for focused research training that will prepare you for your primary area of research.

Once you have decided your primary area, the particular topic needs to be matched to the length of time that you will be in the training program. If you are doing only one year of training, you have time for only a limited project involving the prospective collection of data. Writing a protocol for a major prospective study, putting it through an ethics committee, obtaining grant support, and enrolling patients often takes years. If you have only one year, doing analyses of a previously collected database is probably more feasible. However, if you are doing a PhD and expect to be in the program for three or more years, doing an ambitious prospective research project is appropriate. It should not be a large clinical trial involving thousands of patients, but it would be worthwhile to get experience prospectively collecting your own data.

There are additional considerations when working on a Master's or PhD thesis. For example, a PhD requires an original research contribution. This is typically not required for a Master's degree. Make sure you check all the requirements of your program. Your project needs to provide you with the necessary skills to succeed as a physician-scientist, but you must make sure it fits the program requirements as well.

Many new physician-scientists have trouble early in their career because they have not developed the skills they need to flourish. These skills involve the ability to identify a good research project, to put together a protocol independently, to put the protocol through the ethics committee, to prospectively collect data and analyze it independently, to write papers, and to deal with journals. Your focused training is the time to develop these skills. If you spend all of your time doing secondary data analyses of previously collected data, you will not have the entire skill set required to succeed when you finally become a physician-scientist. Therefore, even at an early stage, be cognizant of the spectrum of skills you will need to succeed. You can get an idea of this spectrum by discussing it with mentors and other junior physician-scientists. They can be helpful in telling you what courses you should take, what projects you should be involved in, and what research skills are in demand. It will be useful for you to be involved in several different kinds of projects during your training so that you can develop different types of skills. By performing an eclectic set of research projects, you will develop an extensive knowledge base about different research methods. At the same time, your primary project should be an in-depth investigation of a particular topic that will provide you with in-depth knowledge of the particular set of skills and tools that will help propel your career as a physician-scientist.

Secondary Research Projects

"Publish or perish" accurately describes the imperative for physician-scientists. You cannot be a successful physician-scientist unless you become skilled at writing and publishing. I will explore the details of writing and publishing in later chapters. However, as a research trainee, you will need to develop good biomedical writing skills. Not only do you need to become an adept writer, but you also need to be productive. If you publish only one or two papers during your time as a research trainee, you will not be an attractive job candidate, and you will not have enough experience to successfully write and publish papers when you become an independent researcher.

It would be optimal to finish your training program with multiple publications. They do not all have to be published at the time you finish, but it is advisable to have several published and several more in press. To have multiple publications, you need to be involved in several different projects. Your primary project will be a large-scale undertaking that may take several years to bring to fruition. However, you should be involved in other projects as well. These projects may be original research projects spearheaded by you or by others. As a result, you will not be first author on all of these publications. Nevertheless, it is useful to get the experience of collaborating as a co-investigator on other researchers' projects. It will also help expand your CV. Importantly, what people look for when reviewing your CV is the number of first author publications you have in high-impact journals. Consequently, it would be ideal if you could generate several publications like this during your training.

Clearly, your primary project should be one of these types of projects. However, it would helpful if you had several secondary projects that would also give you first author publications in good journals. I will go into more detail about this issue in Chapter 10, but make a point of writing several articles in addition to those that result from your primary project during your training. In addition to original research articles, your articles could include meta-analyses, systematic reviews, and editorials. These articles should be written in conjunction with your training supervisor. A systematic review will allow you to review the literature for your primary project and at the same time garner you an early publication. Often, your supervisor will have ideas for articles along these lines. These should not be the primary focus of your research training. However, they can be very helpful. When you have only one or two publications at the completion of your training, you will not be very appealing as a job candidate. In addition, writing multiple articles allows you to develop your biomedical writing skills during your training, so that you are prepared when you begin your first job as a physician-scientist. You need to begin your job search with a strong CV. It should highlight excellent clinical and research training and an excellent publication record. Keep this in mind right from the beginning of your research training program.

What to Avoid During Training

Many paths can lead to a successful career as a physician-scientist, but it is often a single, common pathway that leads to failure. Junior faculty members often find that they are unsuccessful at obtaining grant support and getting articles published. Many new physician-scientists have difficulty setting up a research team and getting a strong research program going. Often, these individuals give up research after several years. Why did these individuals fail? If you ask them, they will say that it was difficult to obtain grant support. They will mention how painful it was to write grants and how competitive it was to obtain funding. This is all true. Frequently, however, these individuals are unable to successfully establish themselves as independent researchers primarily because their research training was inadequate in preparing them for these challenges. I see many individuals who do a year or two of additional clinical/research training. This is not the same as focused research training. These individuals often do not develop the skills they need to succeed as physician-scientists. They may have written several papers that have been published in good quality journals, but they have not developed the skills needed to function as an independent principal investigator.

There are many critical skills to develop during research training. You must learn how to:

(1) Identify feasible and compelling research projects.
(2) Write a protocol.
(3) Get a protocol approved by an ethics committee.
(4) Collect data and analyze it.
(5) Write a good quality original research article.
(6) Get an article published in an expeditious manner.
(7) Write grants.
(8) Manage multiple projects simultaneously.
(9) Mentor junior individuals.
(10) Manage a research team.

It is important to choose a training program that will allow you to develop each of these skills. During the interview process, make certain to discover whether you can be involved in multiple different projects so that you develop the skill set required to succeed as a physician-scientist. Choosing the right research program and the right laboratory mentor is critical.

Summary

To become a successful physician-scientist, you need to obtain focused research training. You likely had excellent clinical training at the medical student, resident, and fellowship level. It is important to do the same when it comes to research training. Do not shortchange yourself. Devote sufficient time to learning the skill set you need in your chosen career. If you are going to become a basic science researcher, you will need to spend years in the laboratory developing the necessary knowledge and skills. This likely involves obtaining a PhD as well as performing post-doctoral work. If you want to become a clinical researcher, you need to spend at least one year developing the knowledge and skills you need for this type of research, and ideally you will pursue a Master's or a PhD degree as well. Be very selective about the program you choose. To identify the research program that is most appropriate for you, interact with mentors and contacts at your current institution and other institutions and talk to individuals at the laboratories you are considering. Interview at multiple laboratories to determine the best match for you. The program you choose is one of the most important determinants of whether you are going to succeed as a physician-scientist.

Key Points

- Obtain excellent focused research training.
- Consult with your mentors, individuals at the institutions you are interested in, and others to get in-depth information about each program.
- Examine websites and publications to get a clear picture of each laboratory.
- Put together a strong personal statement and CV.
- Make sure your publication record is strong.
- Have mentors send reference letters and, if possible, make phone calls on your behalf.
- Carefully consider what you need to find out about an institution before going to an interview.
- Choose a primary research topic that is feasible to accomplish during your training.
- Choose secondary projects that will enable you to publish additional articles and gain additional experience without detracting from your primary project.
- Develop research, writing, and management skills before arriving at your first job.

Suggested Reading

1. Early Career Development Resources. http://www.americanheart.org/presenter.jhtml?identifier=3004039. Accessed July 3, 2009.
2. Faculty Vitae. http://www.aamc.org/members/facultydev/facultyvitae/start.htm. Accessed July 3, 2009.
3. Cope AP, Brennan FM, Hill Gaston JS, Haskard DO. Planning your research training. Rheumatology (Oxford) 2005; 44: 1339–1340.
4. Goldhamer ME, Cohen AP, Bates DW, et al. Protecting an endangered species: training physicians to conduct clinical research. Acad Med 2009; 84: 439–445.

5. Gordon C, Salmon M. Postgraduate degrees for rheumatology trainees: an options appraisal of MD, PhD and MSc degrees. On behalf of the BSR Research and Training Committee. J Rheumatol 1999; 38: 1290–1293.
6. Pickering C. Unique training brings young scientists up to speed in translational research. Dis Model Mech 2009; 2: 211.
7. Wilkinson WE, Oddone EZ. Training physicians for careers in clinical research: a tailored educational experience. Nat Biotechnol 2002; 20: 99–100.

Part II
Launching Your Career
as a Physician-Scientist

Experience is a hard teacher because she gives the test first, the lesson afterward.

–Vernon Law

Chapter 4
Getting a Job

If opportunity doesn't knock, build a door.

–Milton Berle

Introduction

In this chapter, I discuss how to get a job as a physician-scientist. Where can you look for jobs? How do you prepare an academic CV? What should you keep in mind during an interview and while negotiating your start-up package? Although this discussion is directed towards physician-scientists who are just finishing their training and are looking for their first jobs, many of these issues are pertinent to mid-career and senior physician-scientists as well.

When and Where Are the Best Places to Look for Jobs?

It is important to begin your job search well in advance. In most cases, this means approximately one year before your training is finished. Because most medical training is based on the July 1 academic year, begin your search in July of the previous year. New assistant professors typically start in July following the conclusion of their training. For more senior physician-scientists, the timeline is usually shorter than one year. Familiarize yourself with available job search resources well in advance so that you can get a good idea of what is out there and how to best proceed.

Journal Advertisements

There are many places to look for job opportunities. I encourage you to explore all of them simultaneously. One place to begin would be the physician job section of the *New England Journal of Medicine*. These listings can be accessed on their website and in print. Refine your search according to clinical specialty, type of job,

M.J. Eisenberg, *The Physician Scientist's Career Guide*,
DOI 10.1007/978-1-60327-908-6_4, © Springer Science+Business Media, LLC 2011

and geographic location. The majority of jobs posted on sites like the *New England's* are for pure clinicians. Their site will give you a good idea of what types of jobs are available. Carefully examine the descriptions of each job to identify whether they are looking for physician-scientists.

In addition to the *New England Journal of Medicine*, each specialty has one or two journals that post jobs. You can access these jobs either electronically or by obtaining a subscription for a hard copy of the journal. Most job advertisements provide a profile of the type of individual they are looking for. If you are looking for a position as a physician-scientist with 80% protected time for research, do not respond to advertisements that are clearly seeking full-time clinicians.

Mentors

In addition to journal advertisements, discuss your career prospects with mentors you have developed relationships with over the years. Also, have face-to-face meetings with your current training director and laboratory supervisor. Current and past mentors are often in tune with what jobs are available or will become available in the next few years. Many jobs are not advertised; instead, they are filled internally. If these individuals cannot help you, they may have colleagues at other institutions who are aware of jobs. They may also be able to initiate contact on your behalf and recommend you to individuals or institutions that are hiring. Therefore, it is useful to discuss your situation with high-ranking individuals that you know at different institutions. Discuss your job search with senior members of your institution and colleagues you have worked with closely in the past. These discussions should take place well in advance of the date you want to start applying for jobs.

Cold Inquiries

Another route for identifying jobs is to send out a cold inquiry by e-mail or snail mail to institutions that you are interested in working at. Send a cover letter and CV to the department or division chair of the institution. Also, send a copy to the director of their research institute. Be selective about which institutions you send these letters to. Send them only to institutions that you are seriously considering. You may want to contact institutions that have potential collaborators and/or specific equipment relevant to your area of research. Perform internet searches of these institutions before approaching them. Do not waste your time or theirs if their research interests do not correspond with yours. Nevertheless, it is possible that these institutions may want to increase their complement of physician-scientists and their research capacity. If your research interests correspond with their future plans, there might be a potential job opportunity.

Headhunters

Another source for jobs is headhunters. Headhunters are individuals who work for private agencies that place individuals in jobs at different institutions. Headhunters are usually more helpful to mid-career or senior-level physician-scientists. Some agencies specialize in healthcare; some specialize in industry; others specialize in education, etc. If you decide to explore the headhunter route, do some research to identify agencies that specifically deal with healthcare and more particularly with physician-scientists. This is not a particularly useful route for new physician-scientists, but one that you could potentially explore.

Your Training Institutions

Many physician-scientists take their first job at an institution where they obtained their clinical training. This is a logical source of potential job opportunities. Individuals at these institutions know both your clinical and research capabilities. They know you as an individual; you are not a "black box" to them. Often, an individual leaves a training institution to pursue additional research training with the understanding that, at the end of their training, they will seriously explore job opportunities there. Whether or not this was discussed while you were training there, send them an updated CV and a cover letter expressing your interest in potential job opportunities.

At my institution, we sometimes identify cardiology fellows that we want to recruit as assistant professors once they complete additional training at another institution. In that case, in their final year of training as cardiology fellows, we offer to partially subsidize their additional years of training if they commit to returning to our institution. If, at the end of their additional training, they decide not to return, they simply repay the money. If you are interested in returning to your training institution in a faculty position, initiate a discussion with the chief of your division well before you leave for research training.

Best-Case Scenario

Your best-case scenario is receiving multiple job offers. Even if your intent is to return to one of the institutions where you trained, it is still ideal to return with several job offers in hand. This will help your negotiations and potentially upgrade your start-up package. Unless your training is subsidized by your institution with the understanding that you will return to a job there, do not give your home institution a firm commitment that you will return. Instead, tell them you are very interested in returning but that you are also exploring other possibilities.

What to Look for

During your search, be very clear that you are looking for a position as a physician-scientist. When exploring positions on the internet, with headhunters, or with mentors, clearly state that you want to be a physician-scientist with substantial protected time for research. It can be a major waste of time, both for yourself and the institutions involved, when you are unclear about the type of profile you are seeking. A beginning physician-scientist should expect a minimum of 50% protected time for research in the first three years; however, 80% would be optimal. Do not consider a position where you will be spending more than 50% of your time on clinical work with the assumption that you will be able to free up your time for research in the future. Such a position is a nonstarter if you are seriously interested in a career as a physician-scientist. If anything, your time will become less and less protected over the first few years of your career. As a result, obtain in writing exactly what your job responsibilities will be and how much protected time you will have for research. If this is not clearly understood by both parties prior to beginning your job, it is likely that your research career will quickly flounder.

When looking at job possibilities at different institutions, it is important to examine different aspects of the institutions. Will your research career flourish there? Are the laboratory facilities you require present? Will you require certain types of advanced equipment and if so, does this laboratory have access to it? Are the types of collaborators you will need available at the institution? Are there other well-established researchers at the institution? Are there potential mentors? What is the track record of the institution with respect to research? How much infrastructure will be available to help you prepare grants?

If the institution does not have a good track record for young physician-scientists, or if it does not have the equipment or the collaborators you need to succeed, do not explore the position any further. I have seen several promising investigators return with advanced training, only to find that they do not have access to the equipment they needed to do their research. Without access to this equipment, their research careers were unsuccessful. Be very wary of institutions that promise to establish a laboratory or provide you with access to equipment but are not willing to put it in writing along with a firm timeline.

In addition to your research requirements, you also need to explore the clinical aspects of the job. You will need clinical exposure at the institution you are considering. If you have clinical expertise that requires a particular type of equipment or access to particular patients, are they available at that institution? For example, a Veteran Affairs hospital, with its predominantly male population, is not likely to have many patients available for the study of autoimmune diseases, so this may not be the ideal institution for you if that is your area of expertise. If you want to set up a new clinical service at an institution, seriously consider how much time it will require. If, for example, I had returned to my home institution and set up a cardiac catheterization laboratory in addition to starting my research career, I likely would have failed as a physician-scientist. Optimally, accept a job where your clinical situation is organized from the beginning. Spend the bulk of your first years setting up your research team, your laboratory, and getting your projects off the ground.

Other questions need to be addressed during your job search. Is the institution in the right geographical area for you? Is it near your family? Is your spouse going to be happy there? Will your spouse be able to find a job? Are there good schools for your children? These issues need to be identified and discussed in detail before accepting a job.

The Academic CV

Spend sufficient time preparing a thorough and professional academic CV prior to applying for jobs. It is likely that you already have a CV. However, update and revise it for your job search. Emphasize your strengths as a physician-scientist and the various roles you have been involved with (administrator, clinician, researcher, teacher). It also needs to detail your research interests. There are many places where you can see what an effective professional CV looks like. To begin with, collect several CVs from senior members of your institution. In addition, many physician-scientists have their own websites that include their CVs. The following are the sections included in my CV:

1. Identification: This section presents my current coordinates, including address, e-mail address, website, and telephone, fax, and beeper numbers. I also include my date of birth, citizenship, languages spoken, marital status, and number of children.
2. Education: I include my post-secondary education; undergraduate training, medical school training, and graduate degrees. I list my postgraduate training including my residency, fellowship, subspecialty training, and research training. I have a separate section for professional certifications, which includes board certifications and medical licenses.
3. Special honors and awards: This section should include any honors and awards you received during your career. These can be related to research, teaching, clinical activities, etc.
4. Professional activities and administration: This section includes any journals for which I was a reviewer. It is possible that, as a trainee, you were asked to be a peer reviewer for journal articles. If so, include these activities in your CV. I also include a section on funding agencies for which I was a reviewer.
5. Committees: If you have been involved in any committees (e.g., training committee), list them here.
6. Professional and/or learned societies: In this section, list all the professional organizations of which you are a member. Organizations such as the American College of Cardiology, the American Heart Association, the American Medical Association, etc., should be included here.
7. Scientific and professional meetings attended: Many individuals do not include this section, but I find it helpful. List every medical conference you have attended. This demonstrates to potential employers that you are serious about a research career. They can see that you regularly attend different conferences, both research and clinical.

8. Research: I include several subsections under research:

   A. Personal Support or Career Awards: If you received salary support awards as a trainee, include them here. It is possible that you received them to conduct research as a medical student. You may have received additional support to do one or more years of research training. List these awards including the years covered, the amount of the award, and the agency that provided the award.

   B. Research Grants: As a research trainee, you may have received small operating grants. In that case, list them here. In my CV, I put everything in reverse chronological order with the most recent first. For grants, I include the year they were awarded, whether I was the principal investigator or co-investigator; I include the name of the principal investigator, if it was not me; I also include the granting institution, the name of the research project, and the amount of the award. If you have multiple awards, separate them into submissions currently under review, current awards from peer-reviewed agencies and from industry, and expired awards from peer-reviewed agencies and industry.

9. Publications: This is a very important part of your CV. It is likely that you will not have many publications at this stage of your career, but you need to make sure that each one is listed. As opposed to the rest of my CV, I list my publications in chronological order. This way, I do not need to renumber them each time I have a new publication. I leave a space between each publication so that they are distinct to the reader. I also put my name in bold in the author list of each publication so it is easy for a reader to find, and I identify students that I supervised with an asterisk. I separate my publications into peer-reviewed journal articles, task force publications (including guidelines, consensus statements, etc.), research letters, letters to the editor, articles for which I was a collaborator (e.g., I recruited patients), and articles in the lay press. I have separate sections for manuscripts in press, manuscripts submitted, and manuscripts in preparation. Finally, I have sections for abstracts, book chapters, and book reviews.

10. Teaching: This section is divided into teaching within and outside my institution. For my own institution, I divide my teaching according to what level of students I taught; medical, graduate, postgraduate, or continuing medical education students. I list these activities in chronological order with dates, number of students involved, nature of the teaching (small group, lecture, etc.), as well as topic and location. You may also have a separate section for clinical teaching. If you taught medical students, residents, or fellows, list them with the number of hours, the dates, and the nature of the teaching.

11. Research Supervision: At this stage of your career, you may have supervised junior individuals' research projects. These may have been research assistants or medical students. List them in chronological order with their names and degrees. The name of the research project should also be listed.

12. Presentations: Your presentations should be listed in this section. Include dates, topics, and locations. Divide this section into presentations at your institution, presentations at other institutions, and presentations at scientific and professional meetings. Scientific and professional presentations should include abstracts you presented at professional societies. Include the dates, the titles of the abstracts, and the locations. Although you may think this section is redundant with your abstract section, include it anyway. As you become more senior, you will be coauthor on many abstracts where you will not be the presenter. In this section, list only the abstracts that you personally presented. In the abstract section, list all published abstracts on which you were a coauthor.

General Points

I cannot emphasize how important it is that your CV look professional and well organized. The search committee looking at your CV will also be looking at many other CVs. To be competitive in this job market, you need to create as thorough and professional CV as possible. Do not exaggerate your activities or your accomplishments, but at the same time do not minimize them or forget to include them. As your career advances, you will be involved in many different activities. It is important that you document these activities prospectively, since it is very easy to forget them. Have a systematic process to make sure that all your activities and accomplishments are documented as they occur.

Cover Letter

Your cover letter should describe who you are, what your training is, what you are planning on doing, and why you think you would be an asset to the institution you are applying to. In addition, mention where you are located, what you are currently working on, and when you will become available to work. Appending one or two key publications can be an effective way of demonstrating your research productivity. It also may be worthwhile to include names and contact information of specific references in your cover letter, though I would not include reference letters in a cold inquiry.

The Interview Process

Your first job interview can be an anxiety-provoking experience. You need to know what a typical interview experience is like, and prepare yourself as much as possible so that the interviewers perceive you to be an intelligent, personable, promising, and confident young physician-scientist. Before your first interview, spend time thinking about what it is that prospective employers are looking for. They obviously want someone who they think will succeed as a physician-scientist. Therefore, you want to convince them that you are a highly motivated, confident, and responsible self-starter with promising and novel ideas. Demonstrate that you are working in an interesting area, that you have the management skills necessary to put together a research team, that you are a team player, and that you will be an asset to their institution. Always find out as much as you can about the institution and what the interviewers are looking for before the interview, and tailor your presentation to their needs.

Once you are contacted for an interview, begin the preparation process. For some institutions, there may be a preliminary telephone interview before you are invited to visit the institution for an on-site interview. Do some research on the institution and the major individuals involved in research activities before the telephone interview. When scheduling the interview, pick a time and place where you will not be disturbed. Have a notepad and pen ready so that you can jot down notes during the conversation. Prepare a list of questions in advance so that you can maintain the conversation once the interviewers are done presenting the job position.

Do not discuss hard details during the preliminary telephone interview. For example, it is not appropriate to discuss salary at this time. However, it is important to discuss the profile of the individual they are seeking. Do they want an 80% researcher? Do they want a 50% researcher? What type of research infrastructure is available? What is their vision for future research? Is your area a high priority to them? Have they hired any physician-scientists recently? What areas are these individuals working in? These are the types of issues you need to discuss.

Visiting the Institution

When a preliminary telephone interview goes well, you will be invited to visit the institution. In that case, they should pay for your plane fare, hotel, and food. You will typically be asked to come for 1 day. You will probably arrive the night before, interview all day, and leave that evening. Be prepared for a long day. It is essential that you be well rested. Dress professionally. You will probably be asked to give a job talk during the interview.

Job Talk

The job talk is usually 45 minutes long, followed by 10–15 minutes of questions. It is often a deciding factor in an institution's decision to hire you or not, so be very well prepared (Table 4.1). Your talk should focus on your research area. Since most individuals will not be familiar with your research area, a certain amount of background information will be required. Take 10–15 minutes to present the background of your research, followed by highlights of some of your experiments and results. At

Table 4.1 Tips for academic job talks

1. Investigate the format: length, audience, available audio-visual equipment, etc.
2. Attend job talks at your own institution to see what works and what does not
3. Get friends, colleagues, and mentors to ask you tough questions
4. Identify sections that can be skipped if you run out of time
5. Bring a back-up file of your presentation
6. Thank the people who invited you
7. Limit jargon, and define anything you do need to use
8. Give a general introduction if some of the audience are not specialists
9. Use an outline to speak from rather than a script
10. Make a clear connection between everything you say and your objectives
11. Explain the future research potential of your work
12. If you do not understand a question, ask for clarification

1. Boss JM, Eckert SH. Academic scientists at work: The job talk. Science Career Magazine. December 10, 2004.
2. Manuel D. Acing the academic job talk: Marincovich gives pointers. Stanford Online Report. February 3, 2000.

the end, give your general impressions about where your research program is going and what the implications are for the future. Do not give a job talk that does not involve your research. You are being recruited as a physician-scientist, so it is vital that you persuade your audience that your research program is dynamic, exciting, and promising.

Consider your audience and what they are looking for. If you have a project that is about to be published in a high-impact journal, it might be of interest to them. Give them a sneak preview. Be prepared for the possibility that there might not be any questions at the end of your talk. In that case, present questions of your own with additional speculations about where your area of research is going. The job talk is a crucial part of the interview process. Spend a substantial amount of time preparing your slides and soliciting your colleagues for feedback before your talk. Deliver a well-polished presentation, and make sure your slides are informative, clear, concise, and logical.

The Interview

During the interview, you will usually meet with different members of the institution. Some of them will be pure clinicians, others will be physician-scientists, and others will be administrators or staff. Each of them plays an important role. They will provide their comments to the search committee. Be personable, diplomatic, engaged, and enthusiastic with everyone you meet. When you meet with physician-scientists, take the opportunity to find out what they are working on and get their impressions about how their institution is functioning. Is it a supportive institution for your type of research? What were their experiences as junior physician-scientists? Do they have any recommendations for you? Are there potential collaborators for you at this institution? How do they feel about the research infrastructure? Conversations with these individuals will be useful. Spend your time with them efficiently. Demonstrate that you are a promising physician-scientist, and at the same time, seek out information that you can use to help decide whether you want to take a job at that institution.

You will also meet with pure clinicians during the interview. When talking with them, obtain information about the politics of the division. Are there any problems? Are there a sufficient number of clinicians to adequately address the clinical workload? Are they expecting you to spend a substantial amount of time on clinical work? Are some individuals leaving? If so, why? Are they hiring additional individuals? Take the opportunity to discuss the internal structure of the division and how well things are going. If clinicians are not satisfied, it is probably not a great place for you.

You will also meet with the chief. This individual will probably meet with you at the beginning of the day, and will usually be the last person you meet with at the end of the day. Be prepared to give them a summary of what you learned over the course of the day and what you think about the institution and the position. This is a good time to discuss more serious issues. If you were to take this job, what kind of start-up funds would be available? What kind of laboratory facilities would be available? How much secretarial time would you have? Will they guarantee a laboratory technician for three or more years? Will they provide funds for a research assistant for three years? How much protected time would be available for research? Does this understanding apply for three or more years? What will happen if you do not obtain an operating grant and a salary support grant by three years? What will your salary be? What is the salary structure of the division? What would be your appointment? Would you be in a tenure-track position? If not, is there a guarantee that you would obtain one after a certain amount of time? These are the types of questions you need to discuss with the chief.

These are important issues that need to be considered in advance. Do not discuss them in an ad hoc fashion during the interview. Also, do not feel pressured into giving a final answer at that time. Inform the chief that you need to think about it for a week or two. Tell them that you were impressed with the institution, that you are enthusiastic about the job, and that you think your career would thrive there. Nevertheless, do not give your final decision at the end of the day. You need a chance to reflect. You may want to consult with your spouse, a close confidante, and your mentors and colleagues. Optimally, you should have several other job offers before you give them a final decision. This will enable you to negotiate a better start-up package or more protected time.

Interviewing for a job is not a skill that young physician-scientists have much experience with. For this reason, it is helpful to identify in advance the questions that you want answers to. In addition, anticipate the questions that will be asked of you and develop potential responses. It is helpful to have a mock interview or two before your first interview. Similarly, it is helpful to have multiple interviews at different institutions. The more interviews you have, the more experienced you will become. If there is a particular institution that you are really interested in, have one or two interviews at other institutions first, so that you can get a feel for the interview process.

Negotiations

New physician-scientists are not usually experienced at negotiating. For this reason, many of them accept positions or conditions that are less than optimal. It is essential to identify the issues that you want to negotiate in advance. Discuss these issues with your mentors before the interview. The number one issue to be negotiated is the percent of protected research time that you will be granted and for what length of time this is guaranteed. You need a minimum of 50% of your time to be protected for three years, but consider requesting 80% protected time for five years. Protected time is always reduced because of teaching responsibilities, vacations, and administrative responsibilities. If you are promised only 50% protected time, you will most likely end up having less, so arrange to have more protected time than you think you require. If you have 80% protected time, you will be able to get a good start on your research career even if this amount is reduced because of other responsibilities. If you want to have more clinical time in the future, this will be easy to arrange. However, it is very difficult to go from a largely clinical profile to a mostly research profile.

Obtain a firm commitment about how many years your research time will be protected. Most institutions will protect your time for three–five years. If you have not obtained an operating grant and developed a strong research program by that time, you may be obliged to switch to 100% clinical status. It is difficult to set up a laboratory, obtain funding, and produce multiple high quality publications in less than three years. Therefore, be careful of accepting a job where the protected time is not guaranteed for at least three years. With regard to salary, I cannot offer specific recommendations about what you should aim for, because this is specific to the particular position and institution. However, I recommend you discuss any offers you receive with your mentors and ask for their opinion before accepting an offer.

Start-Up Package

The start-up package is very important. Although you need to be reasonable with what you request, you also need to have the necessary prerequisites to get started right away. One of the major issues is space. Space is at a premium in most medical centers. Optimally, during the interview, they will show you the space that you will be occupying. If not, obtain in writing exactly how much space you will be provided. You will need a private office and space for a research assistant and/or a laboratory technician. Ensure that there is sufficient space for the laboratory equipment you will need (e.g., fume hoods, fridges, storage for chemicals). Will renovations be required? If there is anything that needs to be changed or acquired, get it in writing!

You will need access to the equipment and resources required for your research. If the equipment is not readily available, get a firm written commitment to make it available by a certain time. You will also need funding for a half-time secretary and a research assistant to facilitate your research. Remember that it is unlikely that verbal promises will actually materialize. Everything needs to be specified in writing when you accept the job.

In addition to funding for equipment and personnel, you will require start-up funds. While you can apply for some internal funds once you arrive, these will take a while to materialize. In addition, internal funds are competitive. You may not receive them. Obtaining peer-reviewed funding is a process that can take several years. Therefore, it is important that once you arrive at the institution, some discretionary funds be immediately available. These funds can be used to purchase computers, equipment, pay for research nurses, go to conferences, pay a summer student, etc. On top of your other major infrastructure requirements, request a substantial amount of money each year for three–five years. Mentors in your field can be helpful in advising you with respect to how much money to ask for. Do not be bashful! Adequate start-up funds are essential to getting your research program off the ground.

If you have greater requirements because of the nature of your work, such as buying major pieces of equipment, be honest about your financial requirements. If you begin a position with no promise of start-up funds, it will become a difficult situation. Do not put a price tag on start-up funds when you initiate discussions. Instead, present your request to the chief as an open-ended question. Ask how much money is available in start-up funds for your research and for how long. If they ask you how much you need, tell them that you will think about it, because you are not experienced in this area; then ask them how much they are ready to offer. You may be pleasantly surprised. They may offer you more than you would have asked for. Do not commit yourself up front. Consult your mentors about how much you will need. Remember that it may be several years before you procure your first grant.

Summary

Looking for jobs, preparing a CV, interviewing, and negotiating are unfamiliar skills for most new physician-scientists. It is helpful to spend a few hours looking at some of the many books available on these topics. Accepting a job at a particular institution is an important determinant of whether your career will succeed. You may be spending the rest of your career at that institution. It is an extremely important decision and one that you should not take lightly. Hours of preparation will be required before you interview and negotiate your first job. I wish you the best of luck in your search.

Key Points

- Start your job search at least one year before your training is finished.
- Check major journals and subspecialty journals for job postings.
- Make cold inquiries, and speak to mentors, supervisors, headhunters, and training institutions about job opportunities.

- Spend time professionalizing your CV.
- Research the institution you are applying to.
- Discuss the job profile early in the interview process.
- Make sure your job talk suggests future lines of research that you may follow.
- Negotiate a minimum of 50% and preferably 80% protected time for research.
- Negotiate optimal conditions: space, protected time, start-up funds, etc.
- Obtain everything in writing.

Suggested Reading

1. Making the Right Moves: A Practical Guide to Scientific Management for Postdocs and New Faculty. 2nd ed. Research Triangle Park, NC; Chevy Chase, MD: Burroughs Wellcome Fund; Howard Hughes Medical Institute; 2006.
2. Austin RN. Writing the teaching statement. Science Career Magazine. April 14, 2006.
3. Axelrod R. Tips for an academic job talk. PS Politic Science and Politics 1985; 18: 612–613.
4. Fazekas A. How to get a job in academia. Science Career Magazine. September 15, 2006.
5. Gray C. Head-hunting in the health care jungle. CMAJ 2001; 164: 1334.
6. Jensen DG. Tooling up: The dreaded phone interview. Science Career Magazine. March 17, 2006.
7. Melnick A. Transitioning from fellowship to a physician-scientist career track. Am Soc Hematol Education Program Book 2008: 16–22.
8. Mohan-Ram V. Negotiating: Please sir, can I have some more? Science Career Magazine. January 28, 2000.
9. Tai IT. Developing a clinician-scientist career. Clin Invest Med 2008; 31: E300–E301.
10. Taylor RB. Academic Medicine. 1st ed. New York, NY: Springer Science+Business Media; 2006.
11. Varki A, Rosenberg LE. Emerging opportunities and career paths for the young physician-scientist. Nat Med 2002; 8: 437–439.
12. Zemlo TR, Garrison HH, Partridge NC, Ley TJ. The physician-scientist: career issues and challenges at the year 2000. FASEB J 2000; 14: 221–230.

Chapter 5
Appointments, Tenure, Promotions, and Sabbaticals

All our dreams can come true – if we have the courage to pursue them.

–Walt Disney

Introduction

As a physician-scientist, you should have a clear understanding of the difference between a university and a hospital appointment, what tenure means, and how the promotion system works. If you are fortunate enough to work at a university that awards tenure, you should understand what a sabbatical implies. Universities vary regarding their tenure and promotions policies (Table 5.1). As a result, my discussion on these issues will be general. I encourage you to examine the specific policies at your institution.

University and Hospital Appointments

When you first come on staff at an academic medical center, you receive either a university appointment, also known as a geographic full-time university (GFT-U) appointment, or a hospital appointment, also known as a geographic full-time hospital (GFT-H) appointment. In most cases, a university appointment implies that you have obtained a tenure-track position (see below for a discussion of tenure). A tenure-track position will typically allow you to apply for tenure six years after your appointment begins. Thus, if possible, obtain a university appointment rather than a hospital appointment. When applying for your first position, inquire about the possibility of a university appointment. If there are none available, you will receive a hospital appointment instead. At medical centers where these positions exist, however, the most competitive physician-scientists will have university appointments. At other medical centers, both physician-scientists and clinician-educators will have hospital appointments. Most physician-scientists hold GFT-H appointments rather than tenure-track positions.

M.J. Eisenberg, *The Physician Scientist's Career Guide,*
DOI 10.1007/978-1-60327-908-6_5, © Springer Science+Business Media, LLC 2011

Table 5.1 Overview of the promotions process at Harvard, McGill, and Stanford

Title	Maximum time in rank	Promotions criteria	Governing body
Harvard			
Assistant Professor	Three years	• Three years of experience as an MD or PhD with more than one year experience as an instructor • Active participation in teaching, clinical service and/or scholarship	Promotions, Reappointments and Appointments Committee
Associate Professor	Five years or unlimited with tenure	• Excellence and commitment to teaching and clinical service, and/or academic community service	Promotions, Reappointments, and Appointments Committee/ Sub-committee of Professors
Professor	Unlimited with tenure	• International recognition in teaching, clinical service, and/or academic community service	Sub-committee of Professors
McGill			
Assistant Professor	Seven years	• Excellence in one of three categories (teaching, research, and contributions to the University or scholarly communities), generally in teaching	University Tenure Committee
Associate Professor	Five years or unlimited with tenure	• Excellence in two of three categories with reasonable performance in the third	University Statutory Selection Committee
Professor	Five years or unlimited with tenure	• Excellence in two of three academic categories • National and international recognition for scholarship in the field	University Statutory Selection Committee
Stanford			
Assistant Professor	Seven years	• Outstanding performance in research and excellence in teaching and patient care	Associate Dean Review Committee
Associate Professor	Seven years or unlimited with tenure	• Outstanding research nationally and internationally recognized • Excellence in teaching and clinical responsibilities	School of Medicine Appointments and Promotions Committee
Professor	Six years or unlimited with tenure	• Distinguished performance in research, teaching and clinical care nationally and internationally	School of Medicine Appointments and Promotions Committee

1. The Purple Book Appendix 1: Process Charts. http://www.hms.harvard.edu/fa/handbook/purplebook/appointprocesschart.pdf. Accessed March 30, 2010.
2. Clinician Teacher Criteria. http://www.hms.harvard.edu/fa/handbook/purplebook/criteriaclinteach.pdf. Accessed March 29, 2010.
3. Ranks of Academic Staff. http://www.medicine.mcgill.ca/academic/forms/ranks%20of%20academic%20staff.doc. Accessed March 29, 2010.
4. Faculty Handbook, Chapter 2: Appointments and Promotions. http://www.stanford.edu/dept/provost/faculty/policies/handbook/ch2.html. Accessed March 30, 2010.
5. Chapter 2: The Professoriate. http://med.stanford.edu/academicaffairs/handbook/chapt2.html#2.41. Accessed March 29, 2010.

Both GFT-U and GFT-H physician-scientists usually receive appointments as assistant professors when they first start. In general, you can apply to become an associate professor after five–six years and a full professor after an additional five–six years. Although the promotion process is similar for both GFT-U and GFT-H appointees, GFT-U physician-scientists are held to stricter standards regarding research productivity. For GFT-H positions, service to the university, teaching, and administrative activities are given more weight.

Tenure

Receiving tenure means that the university is committed to paying a portion of your salary to protect your time for research for as long as you remain on staff at the university. Obtaining tenure is a highly sought-after goal and is a mark of high distinction. Only a small proportion of physician-scientists are ultimately awarded tenure, in spite of being successful at obtaining grant support and being productive researchers.

Negotiating a Tenure-Track Position

Because of budgetary restrictions, many universities in the United States and Canada have either stopped awarding tenure or have frozen tenure-track positions. When tenure-track positions are available, it is important that you negotiate a tenure-track slot while negotiating your first job. It can be difficult, if not impossible, to obtain a tenure-track position once you have started working. If you do not obtain a tenure-track position, you will not be eligible to apply for tenure. As a result, even if you have been successful at obtaining operating grants, career awards, and publishing articles in high impact journals, you will never be able to obtain tenure. Thus, it is essential to obtain a commitment for a tenure-track position from the beginning, or if tenure-track positions are frozen, as soon as they become available.

Frequently, a newly recruited department chair will negotiate to have a certain number of tenure-track slots as part of their package. If you are considering a move to a new institution, the possibility of a tenure-track slot that will continue to protect your time for research once you receive tenure is an important consideration. If you are a mid-career physician-scientist, you could make your acceptance of a new position conditional on obtaining immediate tenure, even if you do not have tenure at your current institution.

Guidelines and Requirements

If you are successful at obtaining a tenure-track position, review your university's tenure guidelines soon after being appointed. The tenure application is a laborious one, and the evaluation process often takes more than a year. Because you usually have to apply for tenure no later than six years after being placed on tenure-track, it is important to be aware from the beginning of the documentation you will be required to provide. As a result, you will be able to systematically keep track of the necessary documentation as your career progresses.

To receive tenure, you must demonstrate excellence in research in addition to a strong track record in teaching and service to the university and professional organizations. National and international recognition is also required. If your application for tenure is unsuccessful, you might be able to reapply. However, many universities limit the number of times a candidate can apply. Even if you do receive tenure, a sizeable portion of your income will still come from your clinical work and/or grant support. Occasionally, it is possible to negotiate supplemental salary support from your department or division chair.

Tenure-Like Awards

For the many universities that no longer grant tenure, there is often some form of tenure-like award. For example, I know of one university that offers a tenure-like award that is renewable at five-year intervals. This university will pay a portion of the physician-scientists' salaries for as long as they are productive. Productivity is evaluated through a peer review process, and the university renews the commitment to pay that salary component for another five years if the candidate continues to be productive. The advantage of a system like this is that physician-scientists who are no longer productive do not have the guarantee of indefinite salary support.

Physician-Scientists Versus Humanities and Science Professors

Tenure for a physician-scientist is different from tenure for a university professor who is not a physician. Professors in the humanities or sciences join the university staff with appointments as assistant professors. Similar to physician-scientists, they usually have six years to establish their credentials before applying for tenure. Once they receive tenure, the university guarantees their complete salary for the rest of their employment with the university. As opposed to physician-scientists, however, tenured humanities and science professors receive their entire salary from the university. As a result, tenure is essential for them, because their university salary is their only source of income. When humanities and science professors do not obtain tenure, they lose their university appointments and must leave the university.

In contrast, if you are unsuccessful in obtaining tenure as a physician-scientist, your day-to-day life remains largely unchanged. You continue to perform clinical activities, teaching, administration, and research, but your income is totally based on patient-related activities, career awards you obtain, or any supplementation you can negotiate with your division or department chair. The only practical change is that your appointment will change from GFT-U to GFT-H. As you can see, tenure has different meanings for physician-scientists and non-medical university professors.

Likelihood of Obtaining Tenure

The final point I want to make about tenure for physician-scientists is the following: you must be realistic about the likelihood of obtaining tenure. A relatively small proportion of physician-scientists have the necessary credentials to be awarded tenure. In my opinion, the physician-scientists who ultimately receive tenure are those who would continue to do research for the rest of their careers regardless of whether they received tenure or not. In other words, tenure is usually awarded to the physician-scientist who is committed to research whether or not he or she has time protected for it. For individuals who spend only a small proportion of their time doing research or who have limited credentials and productivity, tenure is not a realistic goal. That does not mean that they should not continue to do research.

Tenure is usually awarded to a relatively small number of physician-scientists who are highly productive and spend the majority of their time doing research. If this is not your profile, you should think carefully about whether you want to embark on the tenure-track process. There is no downside to being on a tenure-track. If you are unsuccessful at obtaining tenure, the only practical implications are that you will not have a guarantee that part of your salary will be paid by the university for the remainder of your career, and that you will not be able to take a paid sabbatical. However, your division or department chair may still choose to subsidize your salary so that you can continue to do research.

Promotions

The first appointment you will likely receive will be as an assistant professor. After approximately five–six years, you will be eligible to apply for promotion to associate professor. After an additional five–six years, you will be eligible to apply to become a full professor. To successfully navigate the promotions process, you should be aware of the distinctions between these three levels and of their specific requirements well in advance. In general, the promotions process is similar whether you have a GFT-U or a GFT-H appointment. The three main activities evaluated are teaching, research, and service to the hospital, university, and professional organizations. GFT-U appointees need to demonstrate excellence in research while GFT-H appointees typically need to show excellence in teaching. GFT-H appointees should demonstrate some involvement in research, but this requirement is not nearly as stringent as that for GFT-U appointees. GFT-U appointees are also assessed regarding their regional, national, and international recognition, while this is typically not required of GFT-H appointees.

If you have a GFT-H appointment, there is usually no difference in compensation whether you are an assistant, associate, or full professor. If you have a GFT-U appointment, there may be a modest increase in your university salary once you are promoted. However, regardless of your appointment and salary, there is great prestige attached to being promoted. Therefore, it is essential for you to apply to the next level of promotion as soon as you are eligible and have obtained the necessary credentials.

Assistant to Associate Professor

Promotions are important to your career. However, most new physician-scientists have little knowledge of the promotions process. I was not particularly aware of the importance of promotions. This changed one day when I received a review of a grant proposal that I had submitted. The reviewer's comments were critical. Among them was a comment that I was only an assistant professor even though I had been working at the institution for seven years. The reviewer suggested that something was wrong with me because I had not advanced to the next level. After reviewing the comments, I quickly submitted my application to become associate professor.

The application for promotion from assistant to associate professor has specific requirements. It is sometimes possible to accelerate the process if you have outstanding credentials. Be aware that different institutions have different requirements for promotion to the associate level. Become familiar with the guidelines and the application process at your institution as soon as you are appointed as an assistant professor. In addition, have regular meetings with your chief to determine if you are ready to apply to the next level. When the time comes to apply to become an associate professor, it will be difficult for you to put together a competitive application if you have not kept track of your activities (teaching, research, and administration/service to the university and professional organizations). I will discuss each of these activities in detail in the next three chapters, but I discuss them briefly below in the context of promotion.

Teaching

The promotions committee wants to see that you have been active in teaching at the medical student, resident, and fellow levels, with particular emphasis on medical students. Favorable activities include teaching courses such as physiology or physical diagnosis to medical students. Although teaching medical students, residents, and fellows at the clinical level while on the wards reflects positively on the applicant, it is not viewed as favorably as experience in formal coursework. For GFT-U appointees, teaching graduate and post-doctoral students is also highly valued.

All your teaching activities need to be documented, including dates, times, and number of students. This is important in creating a competitive teaching dossier. Whenever possible, student evaluations should be included in your package. This can be difficult, if not impossible, to collect retrospectively. Therefore, every time you teach a course or a small group session and student reviews are solicited, keep them on file for use when you apply for promotion.

Physician-scientists often spend a great deal of time teaching in an informal manner in the research environment, and these activities can be difficult to document. Names of students, dates they worked, names of their projects and any ensuing publications should be documented. If a student received a grant for summer research, it should be documented. Similarly, if a student published a paper or presented an abstract at a conference, it should also be documented. Promotions committees look favorably on any teaching of medical students in the research sphere. Physician-scientists are often active in teaching in this area, so you should not overlook this type of activity when putting together your promotions application.

Similar information should be collected about research activities with residents and fellows. In addition to the documentation noted above, you should also note the amount of clinical teaching conducted on the wards. For example, if you are an attending on medical wards, this should be documented along with the number of teaching hours. If you taught any procedural skills, you should note the number of hours. Again, I emphasize that promotions committees are more impressed by formal teaching at the medical student level. Although this can be time-consuming and often difficult to commit to as your career advances, it is very important to engage in and document during the first few years of your career.

Research

Research is the second area evaluated by promotions committees. This area is obviously essential for you as a physician-scientist, and you need to be evaluated as excellent in this category. The criteria for evaluating an applicant for promotion in terms of research are the number of publications (prestigious journals are important), the total number of publications as primary author, and the number of publications as senior author. The promotions committee will usually ask for a bibliography of your publications. Publications with multiple authors on which you were a contributing author are not usually given much consideration, and neither are review articles and case reports. Promotions committees want to see original research articles in high impact journals. The committee is interested in whether you are an independent researcher, a principal investigator, a self-starter, and whether you can initiate and complete projects. The committee will also be impressed by your students' publications. Some ask you to place an asterisk by the names of students that you supervised. Again, it is advisable to document this information as it occurs.

In addition to publications, the committee attaches a lot of importance to your ability to obtain grant support. Ideally, you will be consistently funded by operating grants. Inability to obtain continuous grant support is considered unfavorable by the committee. For this reason, you should submit grant applications at regular 6- and 12-month intervals. Make every effort to ensure continuous grant support during your career. The committee also determines if you have been successful at obtaining career awards. Ideally, you should be continuously funded with career awards in the early part of your career. Any period of time during which you have not published articles or received grant support will be scrutinized. Failure to receive an excellent score in the research category will call into question your *raison d'être* as a physician-scientist.

Administration/Service to the University and to Professional Organizations

The third area evaluated by the committee is administration/service to the university and to professional organizations. This area is somewhat ill-defined compared to the previous two areas. The promotions committee wants to see whether a GFT-U applicant is serving on university committees and whether a GFT-H applicant is serving on hospital committees. In addition, involvement with organizations at the state, provincial, national, and international levels is highly regarded by the committee. For example, a cardiologist who is a member of a committee of the American College of Cardiology or the American Heart Association, an applicant who is a member of a practice guidelines statement writing committee, or a physician-scientist actively involved with an organization that raises the stature of their hospital or university would all be regarded as engaging in service relevant to this area. Although it is important for you to be involved in some of these activities for promotion purposes, you must carefully balance your time commitments. If you are strategic, you can be involved in several different hospital and university activities without committing inordinate amounts of your time. This is important because you have to devote as much time as possible to the development of your research activities, especially during the early years of your career.

Submitting Your Application

When submitting an application for promotion, realize that it cannot be accomplished over a weekend. Devote between one and two months to this process. Less time may be required if you have been assiduous in assembling the required documentation over the previous five–six years. If you have not been proactive in collecting these data, more than two months might be required to gather the necessary materials for a competitive application.

Obtain and review copies of several previous successful applications from colleagues at your institution. Most successful applicants are more than willing to share their binders with an aspiring applicant. Reviewing these binders will provide you with valuable information when putting together your own application. Typically, a hospital or university requires a specific format for your documentation, which may differ from the format used in your CV. Therefore, take into account the additional time that you will need to reformat your documentation. Once your application binder is assembled and multiple copies made, submit your application to the promotions committee. It may take months for the committee to reach a decision.

If you are unsuccessful in your first attempt at promotion, you can resubmit your application during the next promotions cycle. However, this is not recommended unless you have substantially improved your credentials. Over the course of their

duties as clinicians at a teaching hospital, most academic physicians develop sufficient credentials for promotion to the associate level. Unfortunately, since there is
no monetary incentive or practical advantage, some GFT-H clinicians never apply
for promotion to the associate professor level. However, I encourage all assistant
professors to apply to the associate professor level. Aside from the prestige associated with the promotion, your division will benefit from having a demonstrably high
rate of promotion. In addition, it is regarded as unusual for an academic physician
with 10 or 15 years' employment at a teaching hospital to remain at the assistant
professor level.

The application to become an associate professor is more difficult for a physician-
scientist who is a GFT-U appointee. Typically, a GFT-U physician applying to
become an associate professor is simultaneously applying for tenure. As a result,
the criteria for promotion are more stringent. Most universities are reluctant to
grant tenure to borderline candidates because of the financial commitment involved.
In contrast, there is usually no financial commitment when a GFT-H appointee
becomes an associate professor. Universities are much more cautious about the number of GFT-U promotions to the associate professor level and are careful to promote
only the candidates with the strongest credentials.

Associate to Full Professor

Associate professors are usually eligible to apply for full professor status after
five–six years. This process can sometimes be accelerated in the case of an exceptional candidate. Review the guidelines at your institution to ascertain if this is
permitted. The criteria for promotion to full professor are similar to those for promotion to associate professor. Although the specific criteria vary from institution
to institution, the following areas are always evaluated: teaching, research, and
administration/service to the university and professional organizations.

For promotion to full professor, you need to demonstrate national and international recognition. This recognition should be documented in a similar fashion as
that used to document your teaching, research, and administration/service activities.
Some of the activities used to demonstrate national and international recognition
include: speaking engagements at institutions outside your city; visiting professor-
ships; service to national and international professional organizations; serving on
guidelines committees and consensus documents committees; serving on steering
committees for international trials; being involved in multicenter collaborations of
national and international scope; and being invited to speak at national and international conferences. All of the above must be documented in the format required by
your institution.

For many applicants seeking a promotion to full professor, demonstration of
national and international recognition can be problematic. Because this criterion is
so important, you need to plan your career so as to have the necessary documentation
ready at the time of your application. For example, to amass speaking engagements

at other institutions, inform your colleagues in other cities and countries that you are interested in coming to speak at their institution.

To become involved at the national or international level, contact organizations such as the American College of Cardiology or the American Heart Association (or the equivalent organizations for your specialty) and volunteer to serve on a committee such as a practice guidelines writing committee. You can also contact a journal and volunteer to review for them. Being a reviewer for grant committees of national organizations such as the National Institutes of Health will have a very positive impact on your chances for promotion. These organizations are continuously seeking volunteers to serve on their grant review committees, and although it may be time-consuming, it is a constructive and beneficial learning experience. It will certainly be helpful in demonstrating your national prominence. You cannot wait until the last minute to organize these types of activities; make a concerted effort to enhance your credentials well in advance. If you remain active in the areas of teaching, research, and administration, and continue to develop national and international recognition, promotion to full professor within five–six years of becoming an associate professor is a realistic goal.

Sabbaticals

Once you have been successful at obtaining tenure, you will be entitled to take a sabbatical every seventh year. In some institutions, the sabbatical can be divided into two six-month periods in succeeding years. Importantly, you will be entitled to receive only your university salary during your sabbatical. If most of your salary comes from clinical work, your income will drop significantly during your sabbatical year.

My Philosophy

In my opinion, your sabbatical should not be a year where you do more of the same. A sabbatical is intended to give you a chance to recharge your batteries and explore new directions in your research. If you are a highly productive researcher who writes many papers, the year should not be spent writing the same types of papers. The idea is to get a new perspective or new approach to a problem. You can learn a new technique or a new skill set. Spend the time doing the things you never seem to have time for at your home institution.

One possibility is to obtain a new degree. There are many Masters' degrees that do not require you to be on-site for the entire time. For example, during my sabbatical, I completed the International Master's in Health Leadership program at McGill. Although I spent the year in Israel, the coursework required me to be in the classroom for only five 2-week sessions over 18 months. All of the reading and writing assignments were done between modules.

Traditional Sabbaticals

If possible, I recommend a traditional sabbatical. A traditional sabbatical implies that you and your family move to a different city and research setting for an entire year. Many people go to another laboratory to learn a new technique or explore a new area of research. Others write a book. These are activities for which you would generally not have enough time during your regular activities.

Non-Traditional Sabbaticals

For many tenured physician-scientists, taking a traditional sabbatical is not feasible. In many cases, your spouse may not be able to leave his or her job for a year. For physician-scientists with large wet laboratories, it can be difficult, if not impossible, to move to a different city for a year and still maintain research productivity. A large wet laboratory with multiple graduate students often requires that you be present physically. Nevertheless, it would be a shame not to take advantage of the opportunity offered by a sabbatical. Some physician-scientists take a sabbatical year and remain in their city. This means they are relieved of all teaching and administration responsibilities for the year. They can then concentrate on their research activities. Other physician-scientists who cannot leave their city for a whole year might go to a laboratory in another city for a few months at a time. This allows them the opportunity to learn new techniques that they can bring back to their laboratory.

Finances

The logistics of moving an entire family to a new city for a year can be quite daunting. For many physician-scientists, going on a sabbatical is not financially or logistically feasible. Because the salary paid by your institution may be small with respect to your overall salary, going on sabbatical can be a financial hit. Unless you have substantial resources to help tide you over or your spouse continues to work in some capacity, it can be difficult to go on a traditional sabbatical. To make it more feasible, you might be able to obtain some financial support from your division or department to supplement the salary that is paid by your university. In addition, grants are sometimes available. For example, Fulbright awards can be obtained to supplement your university salary. At most institutions, there is a department of grants and research awards. If you are contemplating a sabbatical, contact this department to see if there is any means of obtaining supplemental funding.

Maintaining Your Laboratory

Considerable thought must be given to the maintenance of your research laboratory during your sabbatical. As a clinical epidemiologist, much of my work can be done via Internet, e-mail, webcams, and fax. It is now possible to have video teleconferencing on a regular basis with your research team. As a result, close supervision is possible even at a distance. If possible, obtain operating grants that begin before, carry on through, and continue after your sabbatical. You do not want the worry of returning to an unfunded laboratory. The idea of a sabbatical is to "recharge your batteries." This should be a reflective year. You should not devote an inordinate amount of time and attention to the everyday tasks of your laboratory. Make provisions so that your laboratory continues to run smoothly while you are away.

Application for Sabbatical

The application process for a sabbatical is usually quite simple. Typically, the application requires only a few pages describing what you propose to do and where you propose to go. You need to obtain a letter of invitation from your host institution. Most institutions are more than happy to have a visiting professor that they do not have to pay for. All they need to provide is an office, a computer, and an internet connection. Nevertheless, be careful about which institution you are going to and with whom you will be working. Unless you are coming with your own grant, your own project, or a book to write, make sure that you are working with an individual who will be able to spend time with you. It is optimal to come with your own data set or your own project.

Clinical and Family Issues

There are many clinical and family aspects to consider. How easy will it be for you to give up your patients and clinical responsibilities for a year? Do you have a procedural skill that you need to perform regularly in order to maintain your current skill level? Is there a possibility of seeing patients at your host institution? How does your spouse feel about moving for a year? What about your children? Although these issues need to be carefully considered in advance, a sabbatical is an exceptional opportunity that should not be lost.

Summary

Understanding the difference between a university and a hospital appointment, what tenure means, how the promotions process works, and what a sabbatical implies is important for junior physician-scientists. These issues are rarely discussed when you are training as a physician-scientist, but they are important issues for your career. If you do not have a clear understanding of these topics, you will not be adequately prepared when the time comes to apply for your first appointment or for tenure, promotions, and sabbaticals. To obtain tenure or a promotion, to be promoted, detailed documentation of your teaching, research, and administrative activities is required. Be proactive in collecting the documentation during your career or you will have difficulties putting together your promotion and tenure applications when the time comes to apply.

Key Points

- If possible, negotiate a university tenure-track appointment.
- It is difficult to switch to tenure-track once you have a hospital appointment; negotiate it from the beginning.
- Only a small number of individuals obtain tenure.
- Some universities offer renewable tenure-like awards.
- Most physician-scientists begin their careers as assistant professors.
- You can apply to be an associate professor after five–six years as an assistant professor and to be a full professor after an additional five–six years.
- Teaching, research, and contributions to the university/academic community are the three major criteria for promotion.
- National and international recognition is needed for promotion to full professor and for tenure.
- Tenured professors are entitled to a paid sabbatical every seventh year.
- A sabbatical allows you to relinquish your teaching, administrative, and clinical activities for a year to focus on research or to relocate to a new place to learn new skills, collaborate with new people, or undertake a new project.

Suggested Reading

1. Making the Right Moves: A Practical Guide to Scientific Management for Postdocs and New Faculty. 2nd ed. Research Triangle Park, NC; Chevy Chase, MD: Burroughs Wellcome Fund; Howard Hughes Medical Institute; 2006.
2. Recommended institutional regulations on academic freedom and tenure. http://www.aaup.org/AAUP/pubsres/policydocs/contents/RIR.htm. Accessed March 27, 2009.
3. Atasoylu AA, Wright SM, Beasley BW, et al. Promotion criteria for clinician-educators. J Gen Intern Med 2003; 18: 711–716.
4. Benderly BL. Science careers. Support for tenure-track jobs in biomedical sciences. Science 2009; 324: 27.
5. Bernstein E, James T, Bernstein J. Sabbatical programs and the status of academic emergency medicine: a survey. Acad Emerg Med 1999; 6: 932–938.
6. Hart IR. The geographic full-time faculty system is dying: can we save it? Can Med Assoc J 1984; 130: 366–367.
7. Kanter SL. Does the consistent application of criteria for faculty promotion lead to fair decisions? Acad Med 2008; 83: 891–892.
8. Mabrouk PA. Promotion from associate to full professor. Anal Bioanal Chem 2007; 388: 987–991.
9. Vickman L. Sabbatical. Ann Emerg Med 1996; 27: 668–671.
10. Wright SW, Slovis CM. Tenure track in emergency medicine. Ann Emerg Med 1997; 30: 622–625.

Chapter 6
Teaching

A teacher affects eternity; he can never tell where his influence stops.

–Henry Brooks Adams

Introduction

Teaching is an important component of your career as a physician-scientist. Not only is it one of the major requirements for promotion, it is also important as a tool for sharing your love of science with your students. Teaching is rewarding! Developing students' interest in research and providing them with the information and exposure they need to adequately assess their interest in this field is a rewarding experience. This chapter covers various types of teaching and supervisory activities but does not address the mechanics of becoming an effective teacher. It is in your best interests to invest time in developing and improving your teaching style. There are many books and courses with helpful tips, and your Faculty Development Office is an excellent source for workshops.

Teaching Documentation

Every time you participate in a teaching activity, you should record the date, subject, and number of students attending. If there is any formal evaluation of your teaching, keep this information in your teaching folder. It is an important part of the documentation that you need to provide when you submit your application for promotion. When there is no formal evaluation, create your own short questionnaire for students to fill out. Ask them to write letters evaluating your teaching skills for you to keep on file. For promotion at some institutions, you not only need to spend time teaching, you need to demonstrate effective teaching skills. In this case, student evaluations are important testimonials about the quality of your teaching. Make sure your evaluation forms or instructions for letters prompt your students to comment on your effectiveness as a teacher.

M.J. Eisenberg, *The Physician Scientist's Career Guide*,
DOI 10.1007/978-1-60327-908-6_6, © Springer Science+Business Media, LLC 2011

Teaching Opportunities

There are opportunities available for you to teach in many different settings. You can teach at the bedside, in courses, or in small group sessions. When supervising individual students in your laboratory, you can teach them research methods. Opportunities are also available to teach continuing medical education courses, to lead a journal club, or to supervise graduate and postdoctoral students. In each of these situations, remember that, as someone whose career combines research and clinical medicine, you have a unique perspective compared to other teachers. Your students will appreciate this perspective, and you can make a major contribution to medicine by sharing that experience with your students.

Teaching at the Bedside

Whether you are a GFT-U appointee in a tenure-track position or a GFT-H appointee, teaching is critical to promotion. As part of your clinical responsibilities, you will teach medical students, residents, and sub-specialty fellows. With more advanced students, you will spend time supervising their work and encouraging them to put their knowledge into practice rather than directly presenting knowledge to them. There are several approaches to teaching at the bedside, and you may be involved with any or all of them. You may teach a group of students in a clinical teaching unit or during sub-specialty consultations; you may teach individual students or residents in a clinical setting; or you may supervise students during operations or procedures.

Teaching at the bedside is not didactic. Students see a patient, perform a history and physical, write it up, and present it to you. You ask them additional questions, and interview and examine the patient. The students provide a differential diagnosis and management plan, and you provide constructive feedback. You might provide your students with references to the literature, to background information of the disease process, or advise them on management issues. You might show your students how to perform a procedure and then supervise them while they perform it themselves. Practical learning at the bedside is essential for students to become effective clinicians. However, this type of teaching is not sufficient when it comes time for you to apply for a promotion. As a result, while you need to be highly involved in bedside teaching, you should not neglect more formal teaching opportunities.

Teaching Courses

In addition to bedside teaching, you will have many opportunities to teach in formal settings. You should take advantage of these opportunities, but be careful not to take on too much at once. You may be asked to teach a course to medical students or graduate students. Each level of teaching requires a different approach and each has its own advantages and challenges. Many factors differ between courses, including the amount of preparation, the time commitment, and the number of credits a course is worth. When the opportunity to teach a course arises at the beginning of your career, offer to serve as a co-instructor or consider deferring such an offer until your research program is well established. Being responsible for a full course can be very time-consuming. You cannot afford such a time commitment while you are trying to get your research career off the ground. It may be better for you to take on a few lectures as opposed to an entire course.

If you do agree to teach a course, choose one that falls within your area of expertise. For example, a cardiologist might teach a course on cardiac physiology and a clinical epidemiologist might teach a course on evidence-based medicine or clinical epidemiology. Teaching subject matter that you are familiar with reduces your preparation time. You are more likely to be confident lecturing on material you know well, and this will be an asset when you have not yet acquired much teaching experience. You are also likely to be more enthusiastic about the areas you know well, which will make your teaching a more rewarding experience for you and your students.

Avoid taking on large courses since they tend to require more preparation time and the content is usually not as specialized. You can, however, offer to teach a module or section of a course that requires expertise in your area. As a general rule, try to teach smaller focused courses at the undergraduate (by which I mean medical students, not those completing a Bachelor's degree) or graduate level rather than large, general undergraduate courses. It is also worthwhile to explore the possibility of teaching a seminar or leading a conference or small group as part of a larger course. Teaching a course can be a rewarding experience, and it is highly valued by promotion committees. However, the time commitment needs to be weighed against your other responsibilities.

Small Group Sessions

Small group sessions are perhaps the most common formal teaching setting for a beginning physician-scientist. Within the context of large undergraduate medical courses, individual tutors often teach smaller groups of 10–20 students. Take advantage of the opportunity to teach these types of sessions. Among other benefits, you may identify one or two students who want to pursue research projects with you.

You may be asked to teach a group of students in an area related to your research. For example, I teach small group sessions on evidence-based medicine and clinical epidemiology. Usually, the teaching material for these sessions is provided by the course coordinator. I teach areas that I know well and that do not require much preparation time. Because of my background as a physician-scientist, I find that medical students are particularly interested in my perspective on many of the issues covered in small group sessions. You may also be asked to teach small group sessions directly related to your area of clinical interest. As a cardiologist, I am often called upon to do sessions on topics like chest pain, electrocardiograms, and palpitations.

Another common type of small group session takes place within the context of the course on physical diagnosis. This course is a time-intensive commitment in which you meet with small groups of medical students and review different parts of the physical examination. Students practice by examining each other before graduating to examining patients. This type of teaching can be very rewarding, and it is also highly valued by promotion committees.

Research Methods

When it came time to present my first application for promotion, I realized I did not have much of a formal teaching record. Unlike many of my clinician-educator peers, I had not spent much time teaching small group sessions on clinical topics and had only taught the physical diagnosis course a few times. However, I realized that I had spent a substantial amount of time teaching research methods to individual students. This type of teaching was almost always in the context of supervising students' research projects. You should not overlook this type of teaching. Like all your teaching activities, it should be documented so that you can include it in your applications for promotion.

I have supervised many medical students, residents, and fellows on individual research projects. Every summer, I supervise students who come to my laboratory for several months to gain full-time experience. During the year, I supervise students during month-long research electives or on a part-time basis. Sometimes, these students come to me with ideas for research projects, and sometimes they ask me for a project. I meet with them at regular intervals while they are performing the project. I supervise their data collection, analyses, and manuscript preparation. I usually have to go over many drafts of the manuscript before it is ready for submission. Unlike more formal teaching, there is often no feedback process for this type of activity. Unless you document the time spent as you go, it will be difficult to provide this information when you apply for promotion.

It is important to keep track of the students you supervise. In your documentation, include their names and level of education, the titles of their projects, the period of time they spent with you, and the number of hours you spent with them. If a student receives a scholarship, record it and keep a copy of the awarding letter in your teaching file. When one of your students presents their research at a medical students' or residents' research day or at a national or international meeting, document it. When a student publishes an abstract or a paper, your CV should mention this and indicate that you supervised them.

Continuing Medical Education

As a physician-scientist, you will have many opportunities to teach in the context of continuing medical education. Because you perform research, you are at the cutting edge in terms of knowledge generation. Many of your peers will want to hear what you have to say about both your clinical work and your research. You will be asked to give presentations at division rounds, grand rounds, and continuing medical education events. Take advantage of these opportunities. Not only are they good for your teaching file, they also give you a chance to consider your research from a different perspective and share your ideas with others. Feedback from your peers can help generate new research ideas or new ways to think about the data you have collected. You also have the opportunity to see what clinicians are thinking about and which issues are important to them. As a physician-scientist, take advantage of opportunities to speak to large groups of people. This is an important skill to master, and it takes time and effort to become good at it. In addition, teaching continuing medical education sessions is highly valued. It demonstrates that you are an authority in your area. In particular, promotion from assistant to associate professor is usually contingent on state or provincial recognition. Teaching continuing medical education sessions can be particularly helpful in this regard.

Graduate Students

Teaching graduate students is highly valued by promotion committees. You will have the opportunity to supervise Master's, PhD, and postdoctoral students. This is a major time commitment and a serious undertaking. Nevertheless, it can be extremely rewarding. These individuals are highly committed to performing research, and their experience with research is often greater than that of medical students, residents, and fellows.

Since supervising graduate students is time-consuming, be selective about the number and type of graduate students you agree to supervise. If you are acting as primary supervisor, limit the number of students that you supervise, particularly at the beginning of your career. If you are co-supervising, you can supervise more students, although you still need to be careful not to overextend yourself. Supervising a graduate student often involves interacting with them on a weekly basis for a prolonged period of time. However, many of these individuals are extremely smart and productive. They can advance your research agenda if you give them the correct guidance. Since they are writing a thesis, they are closely focused on one of your projects. Although they have more time to spend on data collection and analysis than you do, they still need your methodological background and content knowledge. Between the two of you, you can perform an extremely high-level project. PhD and postdoctoral students require less supervision than Master's students. Nevertheless, consider how much time you have available before you agree to supervise them.

Acting as a primary supervisor for a graduate student entails specific responsibilities that are outlined by the university. Before you agree to serve as a student's primary supervisor, review your university's requirements to make sure you have the time to fulfill them. Do not agree to serve as primary supervisor until you have served as co-supervisor at least once. Being a primary supervisor involves much more responsibility than being a member of a student's thesis committee. You need to critically revise multiple drafts of the student's thesis before it is acceptable. When you are primary supervisor, you need to counsel the student regarding selection of the other committee members. In my experience, a smaller committee is better. However, it is important that between them, the committee members possess knowledge of all areas related to the thesis.

To facilitate scheduling meetings, keep the committee as small as possible while still covering all the bases. The committee should be well balanced, with different members contributing different skills and strengths. For example, if you have subject matter expertise relevant to a clinical research project, you might include a biostatistician and an epidemiologist to supplement your expertise. If it is a basic science project, include two pure PhD scientists, one with specific content knowledge and one with knowledge in a complementary area. It is not helpful to have multiple committee members with the same profile.

In addition to meeting regularly with you, the student may also meet with other committee members if they choose. If they do not, they should provide regular updates to other members of the thesis committee. The primary supervisor is responsible for preparing reports of the student's progress for the department. Familiarize yourself with your university's rules regarding theses so that you can appropriately guide the student. Make sure that the thesis closely follows the timeline you established with the committee. In addition, develop a detailed timeline at the onset to keep the student on track. This should include major milestones; certain elements or chapters that must have a draft completed by a certain date to keep everything on target.

In addition to considering your availability, consider whether you have sufficient office space and technological resources for the student to work effectively and productively. Consider what resources they will need and whether you have the knowledge and time to provide them with that training. Your expectations of their contributions also need to be realistic. Have a frank conversation with them about these expectations at the beginning of your relationship.

Post-Doctoral Students

You may have the opportunity to supervise post-doctoral students; individuals who have obtained their PhD and want to obtain a year or more of additional training. The typical length of a post-doctoral fellowship is two–three years. Some of these students obtain faculty positions, some go into industry, and some remain as permanent research staff without obtaining a faculty appointment. Post-doctoral students are largely independent. They should be able to identify a good research project, design the protocol, collect the data, analyze and interpret the results, and write the manuscript with only modest input from you. A post-doctoral fellowship helps the individual make the transition from student to independent principal investigator. In your laboratory, they should polish the skills they need to succeed in setting up their own research laboratory. A post-doctoral student may act as your laboratory manager. With their extensive experience, they should be able to supervise students, perform peer reviews of articles, and write grants. In addition to being a major benefit to your research team, it can be a pleasure to see a recent PhD student blossom into a full-fledged researcher.

Summary

Teaching is one of the most important activities you will perform as a physician-scientist, and it is a major requirement on which promotions are based. Opportunities are available to teach in many different settings. Due to the substantial time commitments involved, you need to be selective about the number of teaching activities you take on. Because of your many responsibilities, it can be difficult to keep track of your teaching activities. However, it is essential that you keep up-to-date, detailed documentation about your teaching activities. Whether you are teaching university undergraduates, medical students, residents, fellows, graduate students, or post-doctoral fellows, teaching is a demanding and rewarding experience. Make sure that you give it the attention and devotion it deserves. Students will appreciate your unique perspective as a physician-scientist.

Key Points

- Teaching is an essential requirement for promotion.
- It is important to communicate your knowledge and love of science.
- As a physician-scientist, your perspective is unique and valuable to students.
- To improve your teaching skills, seek out books, courses, and Faculty Development Office workshops.
- Record dates, hours, and number of students for all your teaching activities, and be sure to collect student evaluations.
- You can teach at the bedside, courses, small group sessions, and continuing medical education courses.
- You can also teach research methods to individual students in your laboratory, lead a journal club, and supervise graduate and postdoctoral students.
- Get involved in formal teaching activities as well as informal ones.
- Consider the time commitment required before accepting each teaching responsibility.
- Teaching small, focused courses often requires less preparation and is more rewarding for you and your students.

Suggested Reading

1. Supervising graduate medical students in the hospital. Jt Comm Perspect 2001; 21: 8–10.
2. Blane CE, Eder DC, Vine AK. Documentation of teaching for faculty promotion. Acad Radiol 1995; 2: 70–73.
3. Collins J, Smith WL. Promotion based on teaching efforts requires ongoing documentation of scholarly teaching activities. Acad Radiol 2001; 8: 771–776.
4. Hovell MF, Adams MA, Semb G. Teaching research methods to graduate students in public health. Public Health Rep 2008; 123: 248–254.
5. Guidelines for Developing a Teaching Portfolio. http://www.mcgill.ca/files/medicine-academic/AppendixA.pdf. Accessed March 25, 2009.
6. Morton JP. The active review: one final task to end the lecture. Adv Physiol Educ 2007; 31: 236–237.
7. Creating Your Teaching Portfolio. http://www.oecta.on.ca/pdfs/teachingportfolio.pdf. Accessed May 13, 2009.
8. Taylor RB. Basic academic skills: clinical practice, teaching, and scholarship. In: Academic Medicine. 1st ed. New York, NY: Springer; 2006: 118–134.
9. Weston C, Timmermans J. Developing a Teaching Portfolio. http://www.universityaffairs.ca/developing-a-teaching-profile.aspx. Accessed May 13, 2009.

Chapter 7
Administration

I've learned that you shouldn't go through life with a catcher's mitt on both hands. You need to be able to throw something back.

–Maya Angelou

Introduction

Like teaching, involvement in administrative activities is one of the responsibilities of a physician-scientist. These activities are important, because everyone has to share the load in academic medicine. In addition, administrative activities are one of the three main areas that are evaluated at time of promotion. Service to your university, professional organizations, and national and international organizations is especially of interest to promotions committees. However, you need to be very selective when agreeing to take on new administrative activities. During the first few years of your research career, limit your administrative activities to those directly related to research. As a newly minted physician-scientist, you have only a limited amount of time to establish a solid research program, and you need to commit the majority of that time to research. It is easy to become overly involved in administrative activities that are unrelated to research. This is particularly true during the first few years. Individuals in your division and department, who are overextended in terms of committee appointments and administrative responsibilities, may view you as one way of unloading some of their responsibilities.

Types of Administrative Activities

There are a number of different administrative activities that can enhance your chances for promotion. Get involved in moderate amounts of research-related administrative activities at the departmental, institutional, national, and international levels. Do not leave it to the last minute to become involved! It is helpful to begin

M.J. Eisenberg, *The Physician Scientist's Career Guide*,
DOI 10.1007/978-1-60327-908-6_7, © Springer Science+Business Media, LLC 2011

with local and regional contributions to build experience before volunteering for national or international activities.

There are many administrative activities you can be involved with such as: (1) serving as the research director for your training program; (2) participating in hospital and university committees; (3) serving on the institutional review board of your hospital; (4) being involved in the organization of scientific and professional meetings; (5) acting as a peer reviewer for journals; (6) being a member of a journal's editorial review board or editorial board; (7) performing grant reviews as an external or internal reviewer; and (8) serving on committees of national and international organizations. Some of these activities are time-consuming and some are less useful for promotional purposes. It is important to be selective about which activities you become involved with. Since you will be invited to become involved in many activities, it is important to learn how to say "no" in a diplomatic manner.

Departmental/Institutional Activity

Research Director for Your Training Program

One administrative role that does not require a large amount of time but is closely tied to research is that of director of research for the training program in your specialty area. For example, I am the director of clinical research for the cardiology fellowship training program at McGill. My major responsibility is to meet with the cardiology fellows and to make sure that they are involved in research projects that are appropriate to their level. I ensure that they are not taking on projects that are too ambitious and that they appreciate and have access to the resources they need. I make sure that the fellows are teamed up with mentors who have research experience themselves. Appropriate mentors need to have experience writing articles as the first author, as well as experience supervising medical students, residents, and fellows in research projects that ultimately get published. I often restrain fellows from taking on large randomized controlled trials that require years to accomplish. In addition, I organize the delivery of didactic lectures on research design principles. Once a year, I help organize the fellows' research day.

Serving as the director of research for your training program is a useful administrative role for a young physician-scientist. This role gives you a feel for what is going on in your subspecialty area within the entire medical center and university. You are in contact with residents and fellows who may want to do research projects with you. It helps you understand what is and what is not an appropriate project for physicians at different levels of their training. This is a satisfying administrative role, which optimally utilizes your knowledge and skills.

Hospital and University Committees

Serving on committees within your hospital and university may not require an extraordinary amount of time and may be useful to your career. For example, the research institute at your hospital may have a research committee that tracks what is going on in your institution. Meetings for this type of committee can be useful, because you get to interact with other members of the hospital who are involved in research. You get to hear about the research projects that are going on, the obstacles in your institution, and what the current funding climate is like. In addition, a committee like this can give you exposure to mid-career and senior investigators. These contacts can be useful when you want to have a grant proposal reviewed prior to submission. It can also help when you have a particular strategic question that you need an insider's view on. In addition to the research committee, there are numerous other committees that you can become involved in, such as the hospital quality assurance committee, the training program committee, the institutional review board, etc. When evaluating whether you want to serve on a particular hospital or university committee, consider the time commitment, its relevance to your research interests, and how your participation will be viewed when it comes time to apply for promotion.

Institutional Review Board

Young investigators are often asked to become members of the institutional review board of their hospital. These boards review the research protocols for the institution from both an ethical and a scientific perspective. Besides learning how a hospital committee functions, you get a good idea about what excellent and poor protocols look like. You gain an appreciation for the following types of questions: what types of studies are being performed in your hospital? What is the process for getting a protocol approved by the institutional review board? How can you be strategic about putting together a grant application?

Early in your career, I would consider deferring an invitation to become a member of your hospital's institutional review board. The experience is definitely valuable, but the amount of time required can be significant. Review boards meet frequently and can consume a substantial amount of your time. In addition, you have to spend time reviewing all of the protocols prior to the meetings, which is also time-consuming. These commitments will cut into the time you have available to perform research. As a result, although it might be a useful exercise, consider deferring an invitation to join this committee until later in your career.

National/International Activity

Scientific and Professional Meetings

It is always an honor to be invited to participate in the organization of scientific or professional meetings. This activity can be a useful experience from which you learn a lot while simultaneously improving your credentials for promotion. However, be sure that the activities you choose are not too time-consuming and that they are directly related to research activities. Some of the activities that you may be invited to participate in are (1) moderating a session, (2) grading submitted abstracts, (3) organizing a workshop, and (4) organizing a meeting.

Moderating a Session

You may be invited to moderate an oral session. This is worthwhile and not very time-consuming. To moderate an oral session, you sit on the podium during the presentations, introduce each speaker, and make sure that they stay within their time limits. While they are speaking, you jot down a few questions to ask after the presentation. At the end of the presentations, there is usually a question and answer session. If there are not enough questions from the audience, ask the speakers the questions you jotted down during the presentations.

Occasionally, for higher profile sessions, you may need to do some preparatory work. For example, for several years, I served as a moderator for the late-breaking clinical trials session for the Canadian Cardiovascular Congress meeting. Prior to the meeting, we evaluated the abstract submissions to determine which studies would be presented. There were a limited number of slots for presentations, and we needed to make sure that only the highest quality research was presented. We sometimes invited selected colleagues to deliver brief comments after each of the original research presentations. During our preparatory meetings, we discussed which colleagues were experts in each area and who would be appropriate to provide comments.

Grading Abstracts

You may be asked to grade abstracts that have been submitted to national or international meetings. This is a beneficial experience and not overly time-consuming. If you have not been asked, volunteer your services as an abstract grader. You usually have a limited amount of time to review a large number of abstracts. However, you do not have to give comments, so reviews do not take long. After receiving the abstracts, review them in an expeditious manner. After scoring all the abstracts, review them again to ensure that your scoring is consistent. Typically, only a small percentage of the abstracts are accepted for presentation. Usually, the top abstracts are accepted as oral presentations, the next level is accepted for poster presentations, and the rest are rejected. Serving as an abstract grader is a useful experience. It gives you a good idea of the types of research projects being conducted in your area, in addition to exposing you to well-constructed abstracts. This can be a beneficial experience when writing your own abstracts.

Organizing a Workshop

You may be asked to give suggestions about the types of workshops that should be presented at a meeting or to put together a workshop yourself. You can suggest a workshop in your area of interest with you as one of the speakers, as well as some of your colleagues who are knowledgeable in different areas related to the topic. For example, you might suggest a workshop on obesity. You could have speakers who address the epidemiologic, public health, and endocrinologic aspects of obesity, as well as a speaker who discusses the development of pharmaceutical agents to treat obesity. Aside from putting together a brief proposal for the workshop, you are responsible for coordinating presentations by the other speakers and for preparing your own presentation. Organizing a workshop is a high-profile activity that you can learn a lot from without committing too much of your time.

Organizing a Meeting

You are not usually invited to help organize a major scientific meeting until you are at the mid- or senior-level of your career. If asked at the junior level, consider deferring this type of activity until you are more established. There are many logistical issues involved in organizing meetings, and much of your time can be taken up by issues that are not directly related to the research content of the meeting.

Peer Review for Journals

Reviewing manuscripts submitted for publication to a peer-reviewed journal is an important activity for a junior physician-scientist. Because you are submitting manuscripts to these journals, it is also your responsibility to review manuscripts for them. It is also an important aspect of your education as a physician-scientist. By performing manuscript reviews, you get a much clearer idea of what a good journal article looks like and what that journal is looking for. Journal editors are always on the lookout for new reviewers. If you are not already reviewing for a journal, identify one or two journals in your area of interest and contact them by e-mail to let them know that you are available to do reviews. They will be more than happy to accommodate you. For your first article reviews, contact the journal and request permission to show the articles to your mentor. Co-reviewing an article helps you to understand which elements should be included in an article review, while ensuring that the authors get a fair review of their work.

Once you are identified as a reviewer, the journal will send you requests to review manuscripts. If the paper is in your area of interest and you have time to review it, respond immediately in the affirmative. If the paper is not in your area of interest or if you do not have time to review it, inform them immediately. Delaying your response delays the review process for the authors of the submitted manuscript. Manuscripts under review are confidential. You cannot share their content with your colleagues or use it to further your own research.

My reviews are usually one to one and a half single-spaced pages in length. I list the title of the paper and the authors' names. I present a one-paragraph summary of the article, mostly taken directly from the abstract, to give the editor a brief synopsis of the project. This is followed by a short paragraph with my general comments. These comments relate to the big picture of the article. Is this a relevant question? Is there some major issue that precludes the acceptance of the conclusions? Is this a groundbreaking article that is truly novel and significant? Following the general comments section, I have a specific comments section. I present these comments in bullet format. I start with comments about the title, followed by comments about the abstract, the introduction, the methods, the results, the discussion, the references, the tables, and the figures. If the paper is poorly written with grammatical and spelling errors, I point this out and suggest that an editorial review would be useful. I do not list all instances that need editorial improvement. I typically read through a manuscript once and type my comments as I read. If I see inconsistencies in the article, I list them. If I have major questions about the relevance of the topic or the approach, I list them as well. You should not need to spend more than two hours on a review.

In addition to requesting your comments for the authors, journal editors usually request confidential remarks directed to them. This section can be short and is often only two or three sentences. State whether or not you think the paper should be published and why. Explain why it is a particularly relevant and compelling paper or why you think it is low priority. Unlike comments to the authors, which should be very diplomatic, your response to the editors can be fairly blunt. In addition to the comments to the authors and the editors, there may be a grid to fill out. Questions on the grid may include the following: what is the priority for this article? What is the originality of this article? Do you have any conflicts of interest?

Review manuscripts as expeditiously as possible. This speeds up the entire review process. In most cases, manuscripts are rejected and the authors resubmit to another journal. In cases where the paper is accepted with revisions, the authors can begin the revision process. As an author, you will recognize how frustrating it is to wait for months to get a decision about your manuscript.

Editorial Review Boards

As you become more senior, you may be asked to become a member of an editorial review board. An editorial review board is a group of elite reviewers of a journal. These are individuals who have demonstrated that they can perform high-quality reviews of submitted manuscripts in an expeditious manner. It is an honor to be invited to serve as a member of an editorial review board, but it comes at a price. You typically have to agree to review a certain number of manuscripts per year. One of the journals for which I serve on the editorial review board requires that I review between ten and fifteen manuscripts a year. If you are not prepared to review a large number of papers for a journal, do not accept a position on an editorial review board. It is useful to gain in-depth experience doing reviews and seeing what good articles look like and what journals are looking for. It also helps you keep current with the literature and enhances your credentials when it comes time to apply for promotion.

Editorial Boards

The editorial board of a journal is distinct from the editorial review board. Serving on the editorial board of a journal is a distinguished honor. Few physician-scientists serve on one during their careers. You are typically asked to serve on the editorial board by the editor of the journal. For some journals, editorial board members live in the same city as the editor, which is also home base for the journal. Board members usually meet once a week and review the submissions. They evaluate submitted manuscripts, identify reviewers, examine comments from reviewers, and make a final decision about whether or not a manuscript will be accepted for publication. Serving on an editorial board for a journal is a distinguished honor, but it requires a substantial amount of time. It is not an activity that you will be asked to perform as a junior physician-scientist.

Grant Reviews

Performing grant reviews is an important part of your development as a physician-scientist. Junior faculty can begin by reviewing for competitions within their own institutions. There are opportunities to review proposals for pilot studies and student bursaries that provide valuable experience with the review process before moving on to reviewing for external funding agencies.

Funding agencies have both external and internal reviewers. External reviewers send their comments once they have reviewed the grants, but they do not attend the committee meetings. External reviewers are not privy to the details of the committee meetings. Their reviews are used by the internal reviewers at the meetings to help decide which grants should be funded. Internal reviewers review grants at their home institution, and then travel to the granting agency for the committee meeting at which grants are scored and decisions are made about funding.

External Reviewer

Early in your career, you may be asked to serve as an external reviewer for a funding agency. Once you become funded by an agency, many expect you to review grants for them. They will attempt to send you grants in your area of interest. However, because of the limited number of reviewers available and the large numbers of grants submitted, you may sometimes be asked to review grants that are only tangentially related to your specialty. In these cases, comment on the areas of the grant of which you have sufficient knowledge. State plainly that the grant is not perfectly aligned with your area of interest and therefore you will unable to comment on certain sections. Nevertheless, an experienced physician-scientist should be able to review many types of grants and decide whether they are well-written, feasible, involve compelling topics, and whether the budgets are reasonable and well-justified. If a grant is directly related to your area of interest, comment on the substance of the grant itself. Are the proposed methods appropriate? Is the sample size estimated properly? Are the outcomes relevant? Are the suggested experiments feasible? Do the investigators have the required experience to perform the proposed experiments?

Typically, an external review will result in two to three pages of single-spaced comments that are sent to the committee. Your comments should include the title of the grant, the duration, and the amount of funding requested. In addition, provide a brief summary paragraph of the proposed study. This summary can be taken almost directly from the grant application itself. Similar to peer review of manuscripts, the summary is usually followed by one paragraph of general comments in which you highlight the major pros and cons of the grant. You will also include a separate section with specific questions and comments. Remember that these comments will go to the authors of the grant proposal, so be diplomatic. You should provide constructive feedback that the investigators can use to improve the grant on the next submission, if it is not funded during the current competition. If there are sections of the grant that you think are good, sections that are confusing, or areas that have not been developed enough, identify them. If there are limitations that are critical but that have not been addressed, point them out.

Funding agencies always provide specific instructions about how to review their grant applications. For example, they often ask for an evaluation of the originality and feasibility of the proposal and the qualifications of the principal and co-investigators. Sometimes there is a grid to fill out. Carefully review the instructions before you begin your review of the grant.

Reviewers are often asked to grade or score the grant. In my experience, most junior investigators give higher scores than are typically given by internal reviewers or more experienced investigators. Most grants are ultimately graded somewhere in the "good" range. Only a small number of grants are graded as "excellent" or "superior," and a similarly small number are graded "poor." Therefore, proceed carefully when assigning scores to the grants you are reviewing. In addition, it is helpful to review your stack of grants several times to ensure that your scores are consistent.

Internal Reviewer

Serving as an internal reviewer for a peer-reviewed funding agency is a distinguished honor. It is one of the responsibilities of mid-career and senior investigators who are funded by that agency. In general, agencies make an effort to place you on a committee where you are suited to contribute. If you are a basic scientist, it is unlikely that they will place you on a clinical trials committee. Conversely, if you are an epidemiologist, it is unlikely that they will place you on a basic science committee. The time commitment for an internal reviewer is much greater than that for an external reviewer. Internal reviewers generally have to review many grant applications prior to the committee meeting. I have often had to read 10–15 grants in preparation for a committee meeting. In the past, these grants arrived several months before the meeting in several large boxes. More recently, grant proposals are available electronically. The funding agency sends a CD of the applications or arranges access to them via a secure internet website. Begin reviewing the grants as soon as possible, since it often takes many hours per grant to provide a thorough review.

For internal reviewers, there are different responsibilities associated with being the first reviewer, the second reviewer, or the reader for a grant. The first reviewer has the responsibility of presenting the complete grant proposal to the committee, including an overview of the rationale, study design, and major pros and cons. The second reviewer provides comments that have not been addressed by the first reviewer. The reader adds any additional comments that have not been presented by the first and second reviewers.

Committee meetings usually last one to several days. They can be grueling. However, serving on an internal review committee can be extremely rewarding. You are exposed to a number of important issues: which kinds of grant applications are likely to be funded and which are not; what excellent and poor proposals look like; what important sections should be included in your own grants; what are the appropriate lengths of the different sections; what a typical budget looks like; and what a strong group of co-investigators looks like. You also get an idea of how a grant review committee functions, who the members are, how they vote, and how they think about grants.

If you are given the opportunity to serve on an internal review committee as a junior physician-scientist, I strongly suggest you accept it. You can even approach a funding agency and inform them that you are willing to serve in this capacity. Generally, they will not accept new physician-scientists for this type of service because of their lack of experience reviewing grants. Nevertheless, if you have specific relevant content knowledge, they might be interested in enlisting your services.

Committees of National and International Organizations

It is worth your time to serve on committees of national and international organizations related to your area of interest. Many of these organizations have local or state/provincial affiliates where you can become involved in various committees in a variety of different roles. For example, serving on writing committees for guidelines or consensus statements is an instructive activity. In addition to providing you with an opportunity to get to know other colleagues who are leaders in their fields, it gives you a good understanding of how multi-author guideline and consensus statements are created. It helps you learn how to review the literature in a systematic way. Your participation will be an asset when it comes time to apply for promotion. Service on these committees is one of the ways in which you can demonstrate your national and international recognition.

If you have not yet been asked to serve on a committee, send an e-mail to a national or international organization and volunteer your services. Check with them about the types of committees that may accept junior physician-scientists. Remember that committees may not be interested in you because you are still a junior physician-scientist. However, as your career progresses, opportunities will arise. One of the committees on which I served was the Task Force on Clinical Expert Consensus Documents for the American College of Cardiology. This committee decides which consensus documents, sponsored by the American College of Cardiology, will be commissioned. Consensus documents are written on topics that are highly relevant to the current climate in cardiology in North America, but for which there has been too little research to date to produce decisive guideline statements.

The committee meets face-to-face twice a year to discuss the different topics for consensus documents that its members have proposed. Once a topic is chosen, committee members suggest the names of national and international colleagues who might serve on the writing committee. The committee takes pains to ensure that there is diverse geographical representation and a fair balance between male and female members. The committee also tries to balance the writing committee with individuals who may not have as much content knowledge, but who are solid clinicians with a good breadth of experience. In between face-to-face meetings, there is a fair amount of work to do. Once a draft of a consensus document has been assembled by the writing committee, consensus document committee members review it and provide comments. The documents are revised by the writers based on these comments. After revision, the documents are passed on to higher levels of the American College of Cardiology for additional review. Once the document has been approved at all levels, it is published in the *Journal of the American College of Cardiology*.

There are other ways in which you can be involved with professional organizations and societies. For example, you can serve as the president, treasurer, or secretary of an organization. You may be asked to participate on committees that are not directly related to research. Consider deferring service in these capacities until you are at a mid- or senior-level in your career. At the beginning of your career, reserve most of your time for research-related activities. Although you will benefit from involvement in national and international organizations, it should be within the context of research.

How to Say "No"

During your first few years on staff, you will be approached about participating on many hospital and university committees (e.g., the pharmacy committee, the quality assurance committee, search committees for clinical positions). Be very cautious about agreeing to participate in these types of administrative activities. It is much easier to join a committee than it is to quit one! Each of these committees is beneficial to your institution, and your participation will teach you how a committee functions, how to be a good leader, and about the nature of the activities that the committee is involved in. However, you cannot afford substantial time away from your research activities at the beginning of your career. Therefore, I recommend that, during the early stages of your career, you refrain from committee work that requires too much time and that is not directly related to research. Be selective about the activities you commit your time to.

One of the most important skills to develop is the ability to say "no." It is extremely important that you be able to diplomatically refuse requests to participate in committees and other administrative roles. I have seen many young physicians refuse to take on new roles in very undiplomatic ways. It is important that you interact in a collegial way with colleagues at your hospital and institution, as well as nationally and internationally. You will pursue your career for many decades, and it is quite likely that you will interact with these individuals in the future. You do not want to create enemies. When you need to refuse an offer of an administrative role, be diplomatic.

When you are approached to join a hospital or university committee that you do not want to join, discuss the issue with your division chief. Then, return to the individual who has invited you to participate and tell them that you would like to participate, but your division chief informed you that you cannot afford such a time commitment at this point in your career. It is useful to deflect the refusal from yourself to your division chief. Your chief will likely be happy to take on this role, because he or she wants to protect your time for research and clinical activities so that you can succeed as a physician-scientist. You can also discuss these issues with your department head. If your division chief or department head thinks it is a good idea for you to take on this new role, try to negotiate the removal of something else from your list of activities so that you do not become overextended.

Your response to the request is best delivered in person, by telephone, or by an informal e-mail. Do not send a formal letter of refusal or a detailed e-mail outlining all the reasons you cannot participate at this time. Be cordial, appreciative, and informal so that no one becomes offended. I have frequently seen undiplomatic communications circulating between individuals, and this type of approach is counter-productive, unprofessional, and can harm your career. Finally, you can leave open the possibility of participating in that committee several years in the future, once you have obtained a career award or tenure.

Summary

As a physician-scientist, you have a responsibility to devote a portion of your time to administrative activities. There are many administrative activities that will compete for your time. The demands on your time will increase as your career progresses, so be very selective about which activities you choose to participate in. During the early stages of your career, concentrate on activities that are closely related to research. Identify activities that are not time-consuming, that you will learn from, and that will ultimately help you in the promotional process. Focus on activities that will help demonstrate your national and international prominence. Be cognizant of the fact that administration is one of the major areas evaluated when you are considered for promotion.

As you get involved in more and more activities, it can be difficult to keep track of them all. Keep an ongoing record of your different administrative activities with dates and details, so that this information can be presented when you submit your application for promotion. It is difficult to assemble the details of the different activities you were involved in after they have occurred. When evaluating whether to become involved in a new administrative activity, measure it against the following yardsticks: how time-consuming is it? Will it help you advance your research career? Do you have a responsibility to perform this activity? Will you learn from it? Are you interested in this area? And most importantly, will your participation help advance research?

Key Points

- Be involved in moderate amounts of administrative activities at the departmental, institutional, national, and international levels.
- Do not participate in so many activities that your research career will be compromised.
- Consider activities that will interest you and increase your chances for promotion.
- Consider the time commitment of each activity.
- Consider what you will learn from an activity.
- Consider becoming a director of research for your training program.
- Become involved in committees at your own institution.
- Serve on committees for journals, funding agencies, meetings, workshops, and national or international organizations.
- Learn how to diplomatically decline an invitation to participate in an activity.

Suggested Reading

1. Berg J, Shellenbarger T. Finding the right faculty: the important job of the search committee. Nurse Educ 1998; 23: 38–41.
2. Brazeau GA, Dipiro JT, Fincham JE, Boucher BA, Tracy TS. Your role and responsibilities in the manuscript peer review process. Am J Pharm Educ 2008; 72: 69.
3. Byerly WG. Working with the institutional review board. Am J Health Syst Pharm 2009; 66: 176–184.
4. Chalmers J. Guidelines and consensus statements: their use and impact. J Hum Hypertens 1995; 9: 37–40.
5. Dickstein K. The plight of the peer reviewer. Eur Heart J 2002; 23: 172.
6. Pisano ED. Time management 101. Acad Radiol 2001; 8: 768–770.
7. Polak JF. The role of the manuscript reviewer in the peer review process. Am J Roentgenol 1995; 165: 685–688.
8. Sataloff RT. Education for residents, fellows, and graduate students: a call for participation. J Voice 2008; 22: 611.
9. Schwenzer KJ. Practical tips for working effectively with your institutional review board. Respir Care 2008; 53: 1354–1361.
10. Taylor RB. Academic Medicine. 1st ed. New York, NY: Springer Science+Business Media; 2006.

Chapter 8
Research

The way to get started is to quit talking and begin doing.
–Walt Disney

Introduction

When starting your new position as a junior physician-scientist, it is important to begin your research immediately. Since the clock starts ticking as soon as you arrive, you need to jumpstart your research program. In this chapter, I discuss some of the issues you will need to deal with when you begin your career as a physician-scientist. How do you identify your primary research topic? How do you establish a research team? What will be the role of your co-investigators and collaborators? How do you set up your laboratory and office? How can you stay up-to-date in your research and clinical fields? This chapter is not intended to tell you how to do your research; only you can determine that. Rather, it is intended to help you focus on important issues that you need to address right at the beginning of your career.

Identifying a Primary Research Topic

Identifying a primary research topic may be the most important decision you make as a new physician-scientist. It is very important that you identify a research topic that is scientifically relevant, feasible to study, and fundable. The topic should focus on a compelling area of research that will have long-term interest for you and be intriguing to both your clinical and research colleagues.

I cannot emphasize enough how important it is to identify a single compelling and feasible topic of research as soon as possible. Spend time thinking about this and identifying several possible topics. Run these ideas past more experienced physician-scientists. Is one of your ideas particularly compelling? Is it fundable? Is it a suitable avenue of research given your training and background? What is the time frame required to examine this question? What types of resources will you

M.J. Eisenberg, *The Physician Scientist's Career Guide*,
DOI 10.1007/978-1-60327-908-6_8, © Springer Science+Business Media, LLC 2011

need? How much can you accomplish in this area before obtaining your first grant? Is the topic of sufficient scope to last you for five or more years' worth of research and propel you into an associate professor position? Is it too ambitious? Is it not ambitious enough?

Ideally, you will already have identified a primary research topic before you start your new position. In some cases, you will be asked to prepare a grant application before you arrive. In other cases, you will be expected to spend the first few months preparing your first grant application while you set up your laboratory and begin your clinical activities. At the same time, you might be finishing research projects and writing papers from the last year or two of your research training. You will be extremely busy; as a result, it might not be the ideal time for you to reflect on what area of research to explore in the next few years. If possible, consider this issue during your research training before you begin your new position.

Your primary topic should be closely linked to the research you conducted during your last years of training. At the same time, your topic should be distinct from the topic addressed by your training supervisor. You cannot conduct the same research as you did during your last years of training. If you do, reviewers at funding agencies will get the impression that you are not independent from your supervisor. If you want to pursue the same area of research, it is essential to get a letter from your training supervisor indicating that this topic will now be your own independent area of research and that he or she will no longer be pursuing it. This letter can be included in your first few grant applications. It is important that you be perceived as a principal investigator; an independent self-starter who is not dependent on previous senior colleagues.

When contemplating a viable research topic, consider your time frame. Typically, your research time will be protected for the first three–five years. If you do not have an operating grant, several publications, and possibly a career award by the end of that period, your protected time for research might be severely curtailed. As a result, identify a topic that will help you obtain an operating grant within the first one or two years and that will provide you with several publications within three years or so. A large multi-center clinical trial is probably not the appropriate vehicle for a new physician-scientist. Although it might be a long-term project that you could spend part of your time on, I would discourage pursuit of this type of project as your principal area of research. Instead, smaller less ambitious studies that are a natural continuation of your previous research training will be more appropriate. Beginning a registry might be appropriate, for example. Successful completion of this project would enable you to conduct a subsequent clinical trial. A moderate size study where you can immediately begin collecting data without obtaining additional funding is ideal. Obviously, the topic should be tailored to your area of research. You should definitely spend time getting input from more senior colleagues and mentors before making your final decision. Nevertheless, this question needs to be decided quickly once you begin your new position. You cannot afford to spend months exploring different avenues.

Be strategic in your thinking about what your research topic will be. You need to be involved in an area of "hot" research. At the same time, it should not be an area in which you will be "scooped" by established senior investigators before getting your own project off the ground. Identify an area that involves a compelling research question and that is a hot topic. It should be an area in which you have experience and one that you can devote a few years of your time to without too much competition. Do not choose an area of research in which other groups are already established. The likelihood that you will compete with them effectively for research grants and in the race to publish is not great.

Get to work as soon as you arrive. Hit the ground running with a topic in mind and a clear plan for your first 100 days. If you begin your new post in July, plan to submit your first grant application in the fall. If you miss your opportunity to submit in the fall, you may quickly find yourself busy with clinical work and other responsibilities, thereby making it difficult for you to put together a strong grant application in the future.

Secondary Research Topics

As I discuss in detail in Chapter 10, it is important that you have a continuous pipeline of projects and publications. Although you need to identify a major research question during your first few months that will be the major thrust of your laboratory, you also need to get several other smaller projects underway that are shorter term and more likely to result in publications in the next year or two. These projects should be feasible. They should not be contingent on you receiving funding. They should be projects you can start immediately. You might finish a high-impact paper from your research training or supervise a medical student or resident in conducting a systematic review, a meta-analysis, or a small original research project. Work on these activities in parallel with your first grant proposal.

Establishing a Research Team

Establishing your research team should be one of your key activities during your first year or two as a physician-scientist. Dedicate time to thinking about what your research team needs to look like. Do you picture a large or small team? Will your work involve bench research or clinical epidemiology? Whatever your vision, start small. If you are doing bench research, hire a laboratory technician as soon as possible. Speak with senior colleagues about how to identify potential candidates. Inquire whether they know of anyone with the requisite training who is currently available. Other laboratory technicians at your institution may have colleagues or friends who are looking for a position. What qualifications do you need this individual to possess? Do you require them to have experience with grant applications, papers, clinical activities, etc. You will be very busy during your first few years writing grant proposals, finishing papers, being involved in clinical activities, etc. If you do not have a laboratory technician, you will have to perform all the experiments yourself in addition to your other activities. In order to leverage your capabilities, you should identify and hire a qualified laboratory technician as soon as possible.

A qualified research assistant will be a strong addition to your team. A research assistant might have little previous experience in your particular area of research, but if they are intelligent and motivated, you can train them to become a major asset. They may not have the technical skills of a laboratory technician, but they will be able to perform other activities. I have had very good experiences with hiring individuals who had just finished undergraduate or Master's degrees with a science major. These individuals are highly intelligent, highly motivated, and willing to learn. In many cases, they can perform literature searches, prepare tables and figures, write parts of grants, and help identify potential co-investigators for your projects. They can also collect and enter data for your research projects. Hiring a research assistant soon after you accept your first job is essential to your success. It can leverage your abilities so that you can spend more of your time performing value-added activities like writing papers and grant applications. If you cannot afford to hire a full-time research assistant, consider hiring one part-time.

A part-time secretary is also an important addition to your team. A secretary can draft business letters, format articles and grant proposals, screen your mail, and field telephone calls and e-mails. In some cases, they can also perform literature searches and identify background articles for papers and grant proposals. A part-time secretary also helps save your time for value-added activities.

Summer students are often valuable additions to your research team. They are usually available from May through August. Hiring several students full-time for the summer can advance your research program substantially at a modest cost; be selective, however, about whom you hire. Students are often highly motivated, smart, and willing to do mundane tasks in addition to higher-level activities. In addition, some summer students may be willing to continue to work for you on a part-time basis as volunteers or at quite low wages during the school year.

It is important to establish your research team as soon as possible. Even if your team is small, it will make a huge difference in getting your research program off the ground. At a minimum, make sure that you have a laboratory technician and/or a research assistant, as well as a part-time secretary. Try to have one or two summer students as well. Besides helping you get your projects started, your team will motivate you to start new projects and finish old ones. Early establishment of a research team is essential to developing a successful research program. Once the nucleus of your team is established and the papers and grants begin to flow, you can start thinking about expanding it.

Co-Investigators and Collaborators

During your first few months on the job, you will need to write a principal grant application. As part of this application, you will need to identify and enlist strong co-investigators and collaborators. It is a common mistake for junior physician-scientists to submit grant applications with themselves as the only applicant. Although you can submit an outstanding grant application, and although you might have the ability to perform all of the planned research, you do not have much of a track record. You can significantly strengthen your application and enhance your chances of obtaining funding by involving a strong group of co-investigators and collaborators.

What is the difference between a co-investigator and a collaborator? In the grant review process, these terms have very specific meanings. A co-investigator is a co-applicant on your grant proposal who is involved in the conception of the project, data acquisition, data analysis, and drafting the manuscript. They are co-authors of any resulting papers. In contrast, a collaborator is involved in only part of the project and is usually not a co-author on resulting manuscripts. When submitting an application, co-investigators supply CVs and collaborators supply letters of collaboration. The terms co-investigator and collaborator have very specific meanings in the world of grant applications; however, in the general world of research, the terms are often used interchangeably.

There are two common reasons new physician-scientists do not include co-investigators and collaborators on their grant applications. First, they believe that including senior investigators on the application will make it appear that they are not independent principal investigators. Second, if they are at a new institution, they may not have networked enough to identify which individuals would be appropriate to include in the application. Both issues are understandable. As a new physician-scientist, you need to demonstrate that you are indeed independent and that you are a principal investigator in your own right. However, including co-investigators on your application does not weaken the application; rather, it strengthens it. You need to recognize that you do not have exclusive knowledge of your research area and that you will require a multidisciplinary team to best succeed. You might have substantial methodological qualifications and significant knowledge, but the addition of several co-investigators and collaborators will provide broader expertise to your research and help convince the funding agency reviewers that you can successfully complete the proposed research.

Even if you are new to your institution, make it your business early on to identify strong co-investigators and collaborators for your grant applications. Do not wait until the application is completed; enlist these individuals at the start. They can provide you with much-needed help with your application. Most successful research projects are the product of team cooperation. In a successful team, each member has a different and complementary skill set. Each brings different knowledge and abilities to the table. When questions arise that I am unable to answer, co-investigators who possess complementary knowledge are excellent resources. Having co-investigators and collaborators with complementary abilities can substantially enhance your chances of getting your applications funded.

Co-Investigators

Whatever your proposed area of research and whatever the topic of your first grant application, enlist two or three other investigators as co-applicants on your application. These individuals should not be in the same area of research as you.

For example, if you are a rheumatologist conducting a cohort study on patients with lupus, you might want to include a clinical epidemiologist skilled in cohort studies. You may also want to include a biostatistician with expertise in cohort studies and a pharmacologist who is knowledgeable about the medications used to treat lupus. Including a well-balanced group of co-investigators significantly strengthens your application. Always choose experienced researchers. These people should be mid-career or senior investigators. A multidisciplinary group of new physician-scientists is not particularly reassuring to the members of a grant review committee.

Hopefully, you will be working with your co-investigators for years to come. As a result, they should be individuals you can learn from. Do they have previous successful grant applications that you can review? Will they give you detailed comments on the drafts of your proposal? Will they be accessible when you have questions? Are they well published? Are they respected individuals who will be known to the grant review committee members? These are just a few questions to consider when putting together your group of co-investigators. In addition to strengthening your applications, your co-investigators will provide you with much-needed guidance on strategic issues pertaining to grant support and on getting your project off the ground.

When submitting an application, you should be the principal investigator. Your co-investigators are co-applicants and your grant application must include their CVs. They should be willing to accept responsibility for the intellectual content of the application. Their inclusion as co-investigators means that they will be actively involved in the study design, data collection, data analysis, and manuscript preparation. They need to be involved in the entire process. Do not include individuals just to have their names on the application. Include individuals with complementary skills who will enhance the quality of the research produced and who will be involved in every stage of the project.

Collaborators

Collaborators have a different role than co-investigators. Collaborators help with a particular aspect of the study but are not responsible for the project as a whole. Collaborators are usually not involved in the study design, data collection, data analysis, or manuscript preparation. Typically, they provide a particular service that is important to the project but that is not substantial enough to warrant co-authorship. For example, they might be the head of the laboratory where your blood samples will be analyzed. They usually have a lesser degree of involvement in the project than co-investigators. Solicit letters of collaboration from them to include in your application.

One particular type of collaborator that is critical to the success of multi-center studies is the site investigator. Site investigators enroll patients in your multi-center study at each participating hospital. In some cases, site investigators are co-investigators, but in most cases, they are collaborators. Their status depends on their level of involvement in the study. The chief responsibilities of site investigators are to identify patients for the study, make sure that they meet the inclusion/exclusion criteria, obtain consent, and enroll them in the study. Site investigators ensure that patients follow the study protocol. When submitting a proposal for a multi-center registry or clinical trial, it will substantially enhance the strength of your application if you append letters of collaboration from your site investigators. If you intend to perform a multi-center cohort study involving hundreds of patients, you should have multiple letters of collaboration from investigators at different hospitals stating that they are very interested in the project and will actively recruit for your study.

It can take years to establish a strong group of collaborators. Typically, collaborators are interested in your particular research area but do not have the training or the protected time to do the research themselves. By collaborating with you, they can be involved in bigger and better projects than they would have the time or expertise to attempt on their own. As a new investigator, you can call upon friends and colleagues you trained with to provide you with letters of collaboration. They should not provide you with letters with no intent of participating in the study. Rather, you should recruit friends and colleagues who will actively collaborate on the study with you. Then, over the next few years, you can extend your network.

In general, the bigger and more ambitious the study, the more co-investigators and collaborators are involved. If you go to a funding agency with a highly ambitious project, a large budget, and no co-investigators or collaborators, there will be concern about whether you can accomplish the entire project on your own.

Collaboration and Communication

Once your grant proposal is funded, it is important to have regular communication with your co-investigators and collaborators either in person or by phone to discuss the progress of the study. In the case of a multi-center registry or clinical trial, your co-investigators and collaborators might be responsible for recruiting patients at their institutions. With other types of studies, different parts of the study might be conducted at different institutions. For example, patients might be recruited and blood collected at certain centers, while the genetic analyses are done at another center. As the principal investigator, you are responsible for the overall data collection and management of the database, as well as data analysis and manuscript preparation. For this reason, you need to regularly communicate with your co-investigators and collaborators to inform them of the progress of the study and to get feedback from them when issues arise.

As you become more senior, your co-investigators and collaborators might also become more senior. As your areas of interest expand and change, you will need to bring in individuals with different areas of expertise. For example, I am currently becoming more involved in the area of obesity and the metabolic syndrome. I do not have much content knowledge in these areas. Instead, my knowledge is in clinical cardiology and clinical epidemiology. For this reason, I enlisted co-investigators who are endocrinologists, hypertension specialists, and lipid specialists. These individuals are all principal investigators and well-respected researchers in their own right. They do not have my content knowledge and vice versa. Bringing together a team of investigators with complementary skill sets substantially strengthens the grant applications that I submit.

Managing a group of senior-level co-investigators can be challenging. Typically, these individuals are at different institutions and may not even be in the same city. For this reason, much of your interaction will be done through e-mail and telephone conferences. You might go from the beginning to the end of a project without ever meeting your co-investigators face-to-face. In that case, it is important to keep everyone in the information loop. If you are the principal investigator, make sure that your co-investigators are well informed about what is happening at every stage of the process. When I have an idea for a grant proposal, I put together a one-page summary of the idea and circulate it among potential co-investigators. I inquire whether they are interested in participating. If they are, I write a draft of the grant proposal and circulate it for their comments. Once the comments are returned, they are incorporated into the proposal, which is re-circulated before being submitted. Once I receive the review of the proposal from the funding agency, I e-mail the reviews to my co-investigators. If the grant proposal needs to be re-submitted, the process is repeated.

Establishing a group of co-investigators and collaborators with whom you can conduct projects and with whom you are compatible is extremely important. You might be working with these individuals for many years. The quality and quantity of your research can be substantially enhanced by developing a multidisciplinary team of researchers.

Chief Collaborator

It is important early in your career to cultivate a chief collaborator (here I use the term informally. In most cases, this individual is actually a co-investigator). It is difficult to perform research if you have no one to talk to about your ideas and no one to review your manuscripts and grant proposals. You need to have a chief collaborator who you can bounce your ideas off. It can be difficult to identify who your chief collaborator should be. It should be someone with whom you share a research interest but whom you also get along well and can envision having a long-term relationship with. If there is friction at the beginning of the relationship, it is unlikely that the collaboration will stand the test of time.

Your chief collaborator does not need to be at your institution. In fact, it is often beneficial for your chief collaborator to be at another institution. If that individual is at your institution, members of grant review committees may wonder whether you are truly an independent investigator or whether you are dependent on that individual. You must be perceived as being totally independent by granting agencies.

An ideal chief collaborator should have a similar area of interest to yours but a different skill set. My chief collaborator is my wife. I am an interventional cardiologist and a clinical epidemiologist. My wife is an academic internist with a PhD in epidemiology. We both have Masters of Public Health degrees as well. We have had a long and fruitful collaboration in the areas of cardiovascular epidemiology and cardiovascular health services research. My strengths are that I work directly with patients with cardiovascular disorders and have a good idea of the relevant issues in the field. I also have a background in case control studies, cohort studies, meta-analyses, randomized clinical trials, and systematic reviews. My wife is more of a methodologist. She principally works with large administrative databases. She has access to completely different data sets than I do. However, she is less familiar with the clinical issues that are directly relevant to cardiologists. As a result, she helps me with the methodological aspects of some of my studies while I help her with the clinical aspects of some of her studies. Because we have different skill sets, our collaboration has been synergistic. We have been more productive because we have had each other as chief collaborators. Our collaboration has increased the number of grant applications funded, abstracts accepted, and papers published. In addition, it has been very useful to have a confidant with whom we can discuss strategic career issues. We review each other's papers and grant proposals. We help each other with promotion applications. We often review each other's presentations. Clearly, our research relationship has been enhanced by the fact that we live together and often discuss research activities outside the work setting. Nevertheless, for the typical individual, having a chief collaborator will substantially enhance your chances of success as a physician-scientist.

Getting Organized

As a new physician-scientist, it is essential that you set up your research laboratory and office as soon as possible. To do this, you need to be very organized and systematic. It is easy to be overwhelmed by mail, e-mails, memos, and all the other responsibilities you encounter during your first few months. You will need to set up a system to deal with each of these issues. By being organized, you will maximize your time to do creative work. There are many management books available that can help you with time management. I encourage you to read one or two of these books. Below, I describe some of the strategies I use to help streamline my laboratory and office.

Setting Up Your Laboratory

How you set up your laboratory depends on your particular area of research. Whether you are a basic science researcher or a clinical researcher, you will need adequate laboratory space and appropriate equipment. Ideally, you will have arranged this before your arrival. It is essential that you get a written commitment for all your space and equipment requirements during the negotiation process. I have heard many stories of individuals who were promised laboratory space and equipment only to arrive and find that nothing was ready. These individuals lost months while waiting for space to become available and equipment to arrive, which significantly set back their research timetables. Anticipate your space requirements and the equipment you need and arrange all of it in advance. Consult with more senior colleagues when setting up your laboratory. In parallel with setting up your laboratory, I would strongly recommend that you set up or become involved in an existing clinic that is closely related to your research interests. If your research area involves diabetes, for example, establishing a diabetes clinic where you have ready access to large numbers of patients with diabetes will be a major plus. You will significantly enhance your research productivity if your laboratory and clinical activities are closely linked.

Setting Up Your Office

Filing System

You need to set up a filing system as soon as you arrive at your new job. Deal with every piece of paper that crosses your desk only once. Look at it, respond to it, recycle it, or file it. Do not let papers accumulate on your desk. Have a filing system that is easily accessible and comprehensible. File information quickly, and make it easily retrievable. I have several different filing cabinets that are exclusively for my use. One cabinet has a separate file for each of the different manuscripts I am working on as primary author or co-author. I keep these files active until the paper is published. This cabinet includes papers I am supervising for medical students, residents, fellows, and graduate students. This is a very important filing cabinet, and that is why I keep it separate from the others. This is my research pipeline. I keep a close eye on everything in it to make sure that each of my projects is moving along.

In addition to my manuscript files, I have another larger active filing cabinet containing the files that I use on a regular basis. For example, I have a different file for each funding agency I deal with. I have files for my cardiology division, for the Department of Medicine, for the hospital Ethics Committee, and for each of the current studies that I am conducting.

I go through these files two or three times a year. I recycle old documents that are no longer needed. I move documents that need to be saved but are no longer active to a filing cabinet that I have in the outside hall. Approximately once a year, I go through that cabinet. If the documents need to be saved but are no longer active, I have them sent to the hospital archives. They can be kept there indefinitely.

Files containing confidential patient data are kept under lock and key. In my laboratory, I keep these files in a locked cabinet within a locked office. In addition, my office is in the research wing of the hospital, which is also locked and accessible only to employees with key-cards and has an electronic door lock. There are federal regulations regarding the storage of patient records used for research. You need to be aware of these regulations and follow them closely.

Having a systematic filing system that is efficient and accessible is very important for a successful physician-scientist. The quantity of information and documents that cross your desk is enormous. Make sure you set up your filing system as soon as possible after you arrive in your new position.

E-mail

The more senior you become, the more e-mails you will have to deal with. Many can be disposed of quickly. Many are just announcements from your division or department or from funding agencies that you can read quickly and delete. You need to respond to your other e-mails succinctly. Other e-mails you need to respond to succinctly. I suggest that you find a regular time each day to deal with your e-mails. This should not be during your time of key productivity. For example, my best time for thinking and writing is in the morning. Therefore, I try to deal with my e-mails in the late afternoon. I keep all e-mails active in my inbox until I deal with them. Once they are dealt with, I file them so that I can easily retrieve them. For very important e-mails or for documents that are of high relevance, I print them out and file them for added security. I also regularly back up my e-mails. Because I receive scores of e-mails a day, I try to deal with them on a daily basis. I have returned once or twice from vacation without having been in contact by e-mail, and have found it extremely discouraging to deal with hundreds of e-mails. It is best to keep up with them on a regular basis. Most can be dispensed with quickly with a sentence or two, by filing, or by deleting.

Personal Organizer

If you do not have one already, I highly recommend that you obtain a personal organizer. I currently use a Blackberry. As a research trainee or clinical fellow, you generally do not have that much on your schedule. Once you become a new physician-scientist, you will have many meetings, teaching responsibilities, and clinical activities. It can be difficult to keep track of all your different activities without a personal organizer. You may be asked to cover someone on a clinical service three months from now. Unless you have your personal organizer with you, you cannot respond to that individual immediately, and you may not remember your commitment to do this if you do not enter it into your schedule immediately. One advantage of a personal organizer is that you have your schedule with you at all times. In addition, all your data should be backed up on your personal computer. This way, if you lose your organizer, the data is easily retrievable. You can have your secretary do your scheduling and upload it to your organizer. I get all my e-mails on my organizer. I find this very helpful, since I receive many e-mails every day about research-related topics. When I am traveling, I do not want to have to carry a laptop with me to deal with e-mails. With a personal organizer, I can check e-mails on a regular basis and respond immediately to high-priority items. Personal organizers can also be used to maintain your contact list. As a physician-scientist, you will develop relationships with many co-investigators and collaborators. It is important to have their coordinates at your fingertips. As a result, I recommend you obtain a personal organizer if you do not have one already.

Computers

You need to have a systematic filing system for your computer. You need to easily access many documents over the course of your career as a physician-scientist. Many times, you will want to refer back to an article or grant proposal that you previously wrote. You need to be able to lay your hands on these files very quickly. As a result, I recommend you create a local area network for your research team. I have research assistants in four different offices. All our computers are connected to a network. Every individual on my team has access to the network. We can access documents that we are all working on from our own computers. Our filing system is not organized by individual but rather by project. This is important, because there is always a turnover of research assistants. If our documents were filed according to the person who worked on them, it would be difficult to find older files. We have a file for agendas of previous business meetings. We also have a file with passwords for the journals we submit articles to and passwords for research sites where we upload our grant applications. With our local area network, every member of the team has access to all these files. While on sabbatical, I frequently used a software program called LogMeIn that allowed me to remotely access our network.

Most research institutes employ at least one information technology person. Become acquainted with this individual soon after you start your first position. Meet with them as soon as possible and have them help you set up your system. Having a systematic way of filing your documents on your computer as well as a local area network for your research team can be a very effective and time efficient method of communicating with your research team.

Staying Up-to-Date

As a new physician-scientist, you should identify your primary research topic, establish your research team, develop a group of co-investigators and collaborators, and set up your laboratory and office. However, this is not enough. To maximize your productivity, you must remain up-to-date in your research and clinical fields.

Meetings and Conferences

As a junior physician-scientist, it is essential to stay current in your research and clinical fields and to become acquainted with other investigators in related fields. You can do this by attending meetings, especially small meetings, where it is easy to meet and interact with colleagues and potential collaborators. However, be careful not to attend too many of these meetings, since it will limit the time available for you to accomplish your research. It is useful to attend one or two major international research-oriented meetings a year in your specialty or subspecialty areas. It can also be useful to attend one or two regional and national meetings. Presenting your research at these venues is useful because other individuals can get an idea of what you are doing, and they may invite you to collaborate in their research activities. Limit your attendance at non-research-oriented meetings. Although it may be attractive to go to an echocardiography course in Hawaii, it will not further your research career.

Oral Sessions

Attending national and international meetings can be disorienting for a new physician-scientist. These meetings are often large, with thousands of individuals attending. There are often many different conferences and presentations going on concurrently. It can be difficult to identify what presentations you should be attending. Initially, focus on oral sessions in your field of interest. In these sessions, there are often junior investigators presenting their research. It would be ideal to present at these sessions. Attend as many of these sessions as possible. They will provide you with an excellent idea of what other individuals are doing in your area and will often give you ideas for additional projects. Being exposed to other researchers in your discipline will help motivate you to finish the projects you are working on, to start new projects, and to establish collaborations with other researchers at other institutions.

Poster Sessions

It can also be useful for you to attend poster sessions in your area of interest. During poster presentations, there is a defined time during which presenters stand by their posters and field questions about their research. This is an excellent opportunity to get an idea of what is going on in your area of research and to interact directly with other researchers. You can read the poster and then discuss aspects of the research directly with the individual. It is also useful to present this type of poster at national and international meetings. This will give you the opportunity to show what you are doing and to receive immediate input from individuals interested in your research.

What Sessions to Attend

It can be overwhelming to attend a national or international meeting. In my field of cardiology, national and international meetings attract tens of thousands of individuals. There are many different sessions going on simultaneously. At the beginning of my career, I was not sure whether I should attend the major plenary sessions where late-breaking clinical trials are presented, the oral sessions involving my areas of interest, or an area that I did not know much about that would increase my knowledge base.

Be eclectic about what sessions you attend. Your major focus should be on your research, at least during the first few years of your career. Nevertheless, it is exciting to attend the occasional late-breaking clinical trials sessions and enlightening to attend other sessions in areas that you know less about. I encourage you, during these meetings, to write down ideas for projects that pop up in your mind in the middle of a presentation. These ideas will be very useful when you return home. When medical students, residents, and fellows approach you about doing a research project, you will have a list of potential topics readily available.

Avoid trying to attend simultaneous sessions. You may have the urge to attend the first two talks at one oral presentation session and then run across the convention hall to another oral session to catch the last two oral presentations. This often does not work because of timing and can be counterproductive and disruptive. Pick your sessions of interest, go to them, concentrate on them, and get ideas for your research projects.

Attend conferences on a regular basis to recharge your batteries, re-motivate your research, and get new ideas. If you find that a particular conference is not that inspiring, consider going to a different conference more related to your area of interest for the next year or two to get a new slant on your research.

Networking

As you progress to mid- and senior-career, national and international meetings become less important for their presentation content and more important because of their networking potential. Many large multi-center studies hold their steering committee meetings during these meetings. Similarly, national and international organizations often have their committee meetings during these conferences. As early as possible, become involved in some of these high-profile activities.

If you are trying to get your own multi-center project off the ground, a national or international meeting is an ideal time to meet with your site investigators. If you are starting a registry or multi-center trial, arrange to have a breakfast meeting at which co-investigators come together to discuss the protocol. You can also set up face-to-face meetings with your co-investigators to review the research protocol and motivate them to enroll patients. Often, research nurses from collaborating hospitals attend national and international meetings. It is useful to meet with them as well. Bring the coordinator of your research project to meet with their contacts. This is a great way to motivate your research coordinator as well as the research nurses at your other sites.

It is always helpful and fun to meet old friends at these meetings. You can get together for breakfast, lunch, dinner, or drinks. These friends may be colleagues that you trained with during medical school, residency, or fellowship. Most of them will be in practice rather than performing research. They are "in the trenches". Besides catching up and having social time together, you will get an idea of the relevant issues that physicians who spend the bulk of their time doing clinical work are facing.

Definitely take the opportunity to attend these national and international meetings. They are helpful for developing new research ideas. They are also useful avenues for presenting your own research and obtaining feedback from more established investigators. Finally, they offer great opportunities for you to catch up with old friends and make new contacts with other collaborators or potential collaborators.

Staying Informed

As a research trainee, you spent much of your time conducting research projects. You likely had limited contact with individuals outside of your immediate research area. When you begin your career as a new physician-scientist, however, you need to get out of the laboratory and meet different individuals at your institution. Meeting with these individuals is essential to your success as a physician-scientist.

One of the key people you need to meet is the financial officer of your research institute. Ideally, you will have some start-up funds available. These funds will be deposited into an account at the research institute. Meet with your financial officer to understand the mechanics of spending these funds. What are the forms you need to use? What is the time frame for reimbursement? How long does it take to pay an invoice? The answers to these questions are specific to each particular institution. Meet with your financial officer early on to sort out these details.

There is often an executive administrator at the research institute who coordinates grant applications. This individual is important, and you should get to know them early on as a new physician-scientist. They can be very helpful. For example, they may be able to point you to other investigators who will provide you with previous successful grant applications that you can review when preparing your own application. The executive administrator can make sure that you are on the e-mail list of the research institute as well as the lists of the funding agencies relevant to your area of research. Get to know this person as soon as possible after arriving.

Stay informed of regulations concerning your department, university, government, and funding agencies. In the past, your research supervisor dealt with these regulations. As a principal investigator, it is now your responsibility to stay informed and follow the rules. Make sure you receive all relevant e-mails and memos regarding regulations and grant announcements. Identify the different organizations that are relevant to you and contact them or have your secretary contact them to ensure that you are on their mailing lists. This is especially important with respect to funding agencies. Funding agencies periodically issue changes to their grant application processes. In addition, they might issue requests for proposals in particular areas. There may be additional funds available for research in your particular area. Becoming aware of these announcements in a timely manner will allow you to structure some of your projects in such a way that they are more likely to be funded.

Summary

The moment you arrive at your job as a new physician-scientist, the clock starts ticking. Typically, you have three–five years to obtain an operating grant, demonstrate research productivity, and perhaps obtain a career award. The sooner you get started on your research the better. It is easy to get caught up with clinical, teaching, and administrative responsibilities. Instead, focus your attention on high-priority issues. Quickly identify a primary research topic, establish a research team, enlist a strong group of co-investigators and collaborators, set up your laboratory and office, and stay up-to-date in your research and clinical fields. If you do this, your research program will get off to a fast start, and you will have an excellent chance of succeeding as a physician-scientist.

Key Points

- Identify a feasible and fundable primary research topic with major public health, clinical, or scientific impact.
- Discuss your ideas for research topics with senior colleagues and solicit their input.
- Identify a primary research topic that will bring you an operating grant, publications, and possibly a career award within three–five years.
- Start preparing your first grant application as soon as you start your job.
- Have smaller projects on the go at all times for maximal productivity.
- Consider the type of team you want to build and begin establishing it.
- Enlist a strong group of co-investigators and collaborators with complementary knowledge and skill sets.
- Organize your laboratory and office as quickly as possible.
- Attend regular meetings and conferences to stay up-to-date in your research and clinical fields.
- Make early contact with the financial officer and the executive administrator of your institution.
- Remain informed of departmental, university, government, and funding agency regulations.

Suggested Reading

1. Andrade FH. Starting a new lab: developing new techniques and hiring personnel. Physiologist 2008; 51: 188–190.
2. Barker K. At the Helm: A Laboratory Navigator. 1st ed. Cold Spring Harbor, NY: Cold Spring Harbor Laboratory Press; 2002.
3. Boss JM, Eckert SH. Academic scientists at work: where'd my day go? Sci Career Mag 2004.
4. Brand RA, Hannafin JA. The environment of the successful clinician-scientist. Clin Orthop Relat Res 2006; 449: 67–71.

5. Dyrbye LN, Lindor KD, LaRusso NF, Cook DA. Research productivity of graduates from 3 physician-scientist training programs. Am J Med 2008; 121: 1107–1113.
6. Fernald DH, Duclos CW. Enhance your team-based qualitative research. Ann Fam Med 2005; 3: 360–364.
7. McGuire DB. Building and maintaining an interdisciplinary research team. Alzheimer Dis Assoc Disord 1999; 13(Suppl 1): S17–S21.
8. Pisano ED. Time management 101. Acad Radiol 2001; 8: 768–770.
9. Sackett DL. On the determinants of academic success as a clinician-scientist. Clin Invest Med 2001; 24: 94–100.
10. Taylor RB. Academic Medicine. 1st ed. New York, NY: Springer Science+Business Media; 2006.
11. Thabane L, Thomas T, Ye C, Paul J. Posing the research question: not so simple. Can J Anaesth 2009; 56: 71–79.
12. Webb DM. Getting and staying organized. Hosp Top 1992; 70: 44–45.

Part III
Building Your Career
as a Physician-Scientist

Energy and persistence conquer all things.
–Benjamin Franklin

Chapter 9
Writing

By writing much, one learns to write well.

–Robert Southey

Introduction

Without good biomedical writing skills, it is difficult to build a successful career as a physician-scientist. Although being a good writer is natural for some, most of us have to learn this important skill. Biomedical writing is a very specific type of writing. Many of the stylistic methods learned in high school and university are not used in writing for biomedical journals. Thus, early in your career as a physician-scientist, you need to learn the skills of successful biomedical writing. In this chapter, I review some of the general tips I learned while taking two biomedical writing courses as a young physician-scientist. I will also give you some specific tips about how to write an original research article; a skill that is critical for your success as a physician-scientist.

Why Improve Your Biomedical Writing?

There are two practical reasons for improving your biomedical writing skills. First, it is not enough to perform good science. If the science is performed but never published or published in an obscure journal that is not widely read, then the knowledge is largely wasted. Good biomedical writing skills can help you get your article published in a better journal, help the article be clearly understood by your readers, and help persuade other scientists that your findings are convincing. For the rest of your career, you will be submitting manuscripts to biomedical journals. A high-quality journal is unlikely to accept a poorly written manuscript for publication. Even if the science is excellent and the results are novel, a poorly written manuscript is likely to be judged unfavorably by your peer reviewers. Acceptance rates at some of the best journals are well under 10%. These journals are flooded with large numbers of high-quality manuscript submissions. A well-written manuscript significantly enhances

M.J. Eisenberg, *The Physician Scientist's Career Guide*,
DOI 10.1007/978-1-60327-908-6_9, © Springer Science+Business Media, LLC 2011

your chances of acceptance. It is not a good strategy to submit a poorly written manuscript in the hopes that the journal will be interested and will give you a chance to improve the writing during the revision process. Your best bet is always to present your best quality work right from the start.

A second important reason for improving your skills in biomedical writing is that it significantly enhances your chances of obtaining peer-reviewed funding. Physician-scientists need to obtain grant support to continue to do research. The current funding climate is not great; in North America, less than 25% of grant submissions receive funding. However, some individuals consistently have a higher success rate when applying for grant support. Although many factors determine the likelihood of a grant proposal being funded (e.g., novelty and feasibility of the topic, the team of investigators), a highly readable and engaging grant proposal is far more likely to be funded than a poorly written one that is obtuse and difficult to read. The majority of peer reviewers will not be experts in your area. For this reason, you should not use hard-to-understand language or vocabulary that is not widely understood outside your area of expertise. Always keep in mind who will be reading your grant proposals. Use words and sentences that convey your meaning and that can be easily understood by people who do not spend all their working hours in your area of research. It is often difficult for physician-scientists, who spend much of their time thinking about a particular research issue, to describe their research in simple, easily understood terms. Excellent biomedical writing is a critical ability, which helps distinguish consistently funded researchers who are published in the best journals from poorly funded researchers who are not published in those journals.

Why Take a Biomedical Writing Course?

Biomedical writing courses are very useful for the new physician-scientist. Although you may feel that you are too busy to spend time taking a course, I highly recommend that you attend one early in your career. You will apply the lessons you learn throughout the rest of your career. These lessons will make it easier to write good quality articles and winning grant proposals. I took two biomedical writing courses early in my career. The first was during my MPH at the Harvard School of Public Health, and the second was when I was a research fellow at the Cardiovascular Research Institute at the University of California at San Francisco.

Harvard

In this course, we presented our work at weekly seminars. Each individual presented a draft of one of their papers, and the other students offered critical feedback. Having your work reviewed by your peers, in person and in writing, makes you concentrate on the quality of your writing. The critiques I received during those seminars substantially improved the quality of my biomedical writing. In addition, it was very useful to see the writing styles of others. It is unusual for us to analyze the elements of a journal article that make it confusing versus clear and convincing. A course that focuses on the writing style of the article rather than its substance can be very effective in improving your biomedical writing and improving your chances of publication.

University of California

The biomedical writing course I took at UCSF was transformative in my career as a physician-scientist. Mimi Zeiger, a well-recognized authority in the area of biomedical writing, taught the course. I highly recommend her book, *Essentials of Writing Biomedical Research Papers*. Mimi has devoted much of her professional life to educating physician-scientists about how to improve their biomedical writing. During her course, I learned many writing tips that I had never previously considered, though once I heard them, I realized they made a lot of sense. I incorporated many of these tips into my biomedical writing, and I continue to use them to this day. I strongly recommend that any beginning physician-scientist try out the stylistic devices suggested in her book. Below, I describe some of the important points I learned from her.

Avoid Synonyms

English is not the first language of many of the people who read your research papers. For this reason, you should not use multiple different words to describe the same thing. A reader whose first language is not English will think that the use of synonyms has a reason, not that it is a stylistic choice to "liven up" your writing. Therefore, it is important to use simple language and consistent terminology.

Use Parallel Structure and Phrasing

Use parallel structure in all of your biomedical writing, including original research articles and grant proposals. For example, if your project has three objectives, you should list them in a logical order in the Introduction. In later sections, present information corresponding to each objective in the same order, clearly identifying the objective to which the information relates. Similarly, listed items should appear in the same logical order (i.e., alphabetical, chronological, etc.) each time they are mentioned. Structuring your work in this organized way makes it easier for readers to follow your logic.

Use Short Sentences and Paragraphs

Use short sentences and short paragraphs in your writing. Mimi Zeiger suggests that, on average, no sentence should be greater than 22 words. Once you start counting the words in each sentence, you will quickly realize that many of your sentences are too long. By the time a reader finishes reading a long sentence, he or she has forgotten the beginning. Similarly, it is very difficult for someone to read a paper or a grant proposal that contains a full-page paragraph. I see this frequently when serving on grant review committees. Even veteran physician-scientists produce grant proposals with single paragraphs, a page or more long, very densely populated with unfamiliar vocabulary and in very small font. If you present a reviewer with a dense text like this, it is extremely unlikely that they will read your text in detail. Now imagine that the reviewer is not an expert in your field and consider how difficult it will be to maintain their interest if your proposal is difficult to read. If you want a reviewer to read your manuscript or grant proposal, present it in the most legible and attractive way possible.

General Lessons

The above are just a few of the general lessons I learned from the courses I took in biomedical writing. There are many more simple and practical tips that can be easily incorporated into your writing. To learn these important tips, you can attend a biomedical writing course or read a book on biomedical writing. The courses that I took early in my career as a physician-scientist were transformative, and I use the principles I learned virtually every day. This cannot be said of many courses. Thus, although I know it is very difficult for physician-scientists to pull themselves away from the laboratory for even an hour a week, I highly recommend that you do so to take a biomedical writing course early in your career. Whether you are writing an abstract, an original research article, or a grant proposal, good biomedical writing is an essential skill that you need to master.

Writing an Original Research Article

Writing an excellent original research article may be the single most important skill to master as you begin your career as a physician-scientist. Below, I discuss several tips that may help you write first drafts and improve the overall quality of your papers.

First Draft

Completing the first draft is often the most difficult part of writing an original research article. Facing an empty piece of paper or staring at an empty computer screen can be very daunting. It is important to get some thoughts down on paper so that you have something to build on. It may need to change substantially, but once you have written a first draft, it can easily be edited by hand or on your computer by using the "track changes" function in Word. There are three techniques that I find helpful when writing a first draft.

First, create an outline before you start writing. This will help you organize your thoughts and consider how best to structure the information you want to include. Prior to writing this book, I developed an extensive outline of all the chapters and sub-sections I thought should be included in each chapter. For each sub-section, I listed specific points I wanted to develop further. While writing the first draft of a chapter, I followed my chapter outline and developed each of the sub-topics that I listed for the chapter. This way, I covered everything I wanted to discuss. Once I composed a first draft, I could re-arrange the text, improve the grammar and the punctuation, and add additional details. I highly recommend that you follow an outline to help formulate your thoughts as you write.

A second technique I find effective is to dictate my first draft. For example, I dictated the first draft of this chapter while lying on a La-Z-Boy in my apartment in Jerusalem while on sabbatical. I recognized that much of what I dictated would have to be altered, much would be edited out completely, and some elaboration would be required. Nevertheless, dictating a first draft gets your basic ideas on paper in a typewritten format, which can then be edited and expanded much more easily. For many people, it is much easier to dictate a paragraph than it is to write one down de novo. Most of us think much faster than we can type, but we can dictate almost as fast as we can think. I find it useful to get my thoughts down on paper as quickly as possible, without having to worry if they are ungrammatical and incomplete or if they flow logically from each other.

I go through many subsequent drafts before I am happy with the final result, but dictating a first draft gives me a strong starting point from which to work. I am not concerned with making my sentence structure and organization perfect; I merely want to create a framework of my ideas from which I can build the final result. If you do choose to dictate your first drafts, I recommend using some type of voice recognition software such as Dragon®. This software recognizes what I dictate and types it out on my computer. Although I find that the transcription is only about 85% accurate, I e-mail it and the voice file to my assistant for editing and formatting. I then have a nice, clean first draft that is easy for me to revise.

A final technique for composing a first draft is to prepare a PowerPoint presentation of your topic. You can present it to your research group and record your presentation. A secretary or research assistant can transcribe the recording, and your first draft will be done!

General Stylistic Tips

Throughout my career, I have consistently used the same format in terms of both the layout of the paper and the structure of my writing when writing research articles. Using a template reduces much of the creative tension that inevitably accompanies writing a new article. I will discuss the format of individual manuscript sections later in this chapter. This section addresses some stylistic elements that apply to the whole manuscript, including the size of fonts and margins and the organization of your paragraphs. Though some journals require things to be arranged differently, using a template to create your first draft is still very useful. Once you are polishing the article, you can worry about journal-specific guidelines.

The manuscript should be numbered starting from the title page. The entire manuscript should be in 12-point Times New Roman or 10-point Arial font, or another font that is accepted by publishers. There should be at least a 1-inch margin at each side of the page. I use a 1-inch margin at the top and bottom and a 1.25-inch margin on the left and right. The manuscript should be double-spaced throughout; a requirement of virtually all journals. A useful rule of thumb is that double-spaced typewritten text in 12-point Times New Roman has approximately 250 words per page.

Make sure that the first line of each paragraph of your article is a topic sentence that tells the reader what the paragraph will discuss. For example, a topic sentence might be the following: "In order to see whether these results were robust, we performed a number of sensitivity analyses." This indicates to the reader that the entire paragraph will deal with sensitivity analyses and will confirm or refute the assertion that your results were robust.

At the conclusion of each paragraph, a summary sentence should clearly restate the major points and conclusions of the preceding paragraph. This sentence is often followed by a transitional sentence linking this paragraph to the next. The transitional sentence can be either the final sentence in the paragraph or the first sentence of the subsequent paragraph. I read many research articles in which the connection between consecutive paragraphs is not apparent. Strive to have a coherent narrative throughout your paper so that the reader understands where you are coming from and how it connects to where you are going.

In addition to following the same general structural and formatting rules in each new manuscript, I also follow roughly the same layout for each section of the paper. I try to keep to a format that is professional and easy to adapt to the requirements of most journals. I want readers to be able to follow the narrative thread of the discussion, so I stick to a formula that makes the information flow nicely from the previous section into the subsequent section. In the following sections, I describe my recipe for a well-written manuscript.

Title Page

The first page of the article is always the title page. I put the title in bold, in a slightly larger font than the rest of the article, at the top of the page. My titles are short and descriptive. Most journals do not use declarative titles giving the results of the study. They certainly do not use questions as titles for original research articles. Just under the title, I include a short title that can be used as a header when the article is published. The authors' names are placed in the middle of the page with their affiliations below. At the bottom of the page, place your address (as the address for correspondence), with all of your important coordinates. Also, include a word count for the article. Some journals require a list of three to five key words to be listed at the bottom of the title page. Others require it later.

Abbreviations

The second page is a list of abbreviations used in the article. Not all journals require this as a separate page, but it can be easily removed if they do not. The use of abbreviations throughout your article reduces the word count – something that editors really appreciate – while the list of abbreviations makes you look organized.

Structured Abstract

The third page is the structured abstract. Generally, the structured abstract should be no more than 250 words, so that it fits on a single double-spaced page. The following sections should be included: background, methods, results, and conclusions. It should give a reader a brief but comprehensive overview of the article.

Condensed Abstract and Key Words

The fourth page contains the condensed abstract and key words. A condensed abstract can be truncated from the structured abstract and should be no more than 100 words. It is a single paragraph, double-spaced. Some journals require a condensed abstract and others do not. I always compose both a structured and a condensed abstract. It helps me gather my thoughts and also improves the organization of the paper, even if it is not required by the journal. In addition, even if I am submitting the manuscript to a journal that does not require a condensed abstract, it may be rejected by this journal and ultimately be accepted by one that does require it. It is much easier to write the condensed abstract when you are writing the rest of the paper than to write it months later. Below the condensed abstract, list the key words for the article. The key words are usually 5–10 of the critical words or phrases used in the paper. For example, if your article is a meta-analysis of drug-eluting stents, key words might include the following: drug-eluting stents, meta-analysis, stents, and stent thrombosis. When deciding on your key words, think about terms that will help readers locate your article during a Medline search of a related topic.

Structure of the Text

In the biomedical writing course I took with Mimi Zeiger, she suggested thinking of the structure of an original research article as an hourglass shape. The opening line of the introduction should be broad and general. The Introduction should become increasingly focused until there is a single, clearly elucidated research question at the end. This single question is the narrow part of the hourglass. The Methods and Results sections are also narrow. They report details of the study and do not discuss the study's context. In the Discussion section, the hourglass begins to open up again. The beginning of the discussion should have a single, clear answer to the research question. Then, the discussion gradually widens in scope and reaches a more general conclusion that puts the research findings in context. There is room for speculation on the relevance of the findings to other areas and for suggestions about directions for further research. The hourglass shape is a useful model when structuring the text for original research articles.

An experienced reviewer can quickly assess the general quality of your manuscript in terms of format, structure, and organization without reading the sections in detail. Experienced researchers submit professional-looking manuscripts, and you need to do the same. Experienced reviewers expect to see separate, attractively formatted pages for the title, abbreviations, structured abstract, and condensed abstract, and they also expect a manuscript to be well proportioned. Reviewers will often examine the proportions of the text before beginning to read it. They recognize that most journals will only publish papers that include 12–16 pages of double-spaced text (introduction through discussion). With this limitation, a maximum of 1–2 pages can be devoted to introduction, 4–5 to methods, 3–4 to results, and 4–5 to discussion. These guidelines are somewhat flexible, but if your paper does not approximately conform to these proportions, an experienced reviewer will recognize it immediately and will have concerns about whether the text is structured in a clear and comprehensive manner.

Introduction

On page five of the manuscript, I actually begin the text of the article with an introduction. The introduction does not need to be long. It can be anywhere from one-quarter of a page to two pages of double-spaced text. I rarely use two pages. My introductions are usually one-quarter to one-half a page. In my opinion, much of the information presented in the introductions of original research articles actually belongs in the discussion. I try to follow the hourglass format when writing introductions. The first sentence should be a topic sentence that gives the reader a clear idea of what the rest of the article is about. The topic sentence can be followed by several lines of background, which are crucial for the reader to understand before the research problem is presented. In the final sentence, I state the research question I want to answer.

Methods

The Methods section is often the easiest to write. It delineates the methods used to answer your research question. I find it helpful to use subtitles such as

"Patient Population", "Sample Size", "Experimental Intervention", and "Statistical Analysis" within this section. If a journal does not require subtitles, you can remove them before submitting the manuscript. Nevertheless, I recommend using them while writing this section to help you organize your thoughts.

You need to structure this section into individual paragraphs that address different but interconnected issues. The topics of these paragraphs vary depending on your area of research. In a clinical research article, the first paragraph often describes the patient population studied, including the total population from which the sample is drawn, as well as the inclusion and exclusion criteria. In a basic science article, describe the type and number of animals you used. The details included in the Methods section should enable readers to replicate your results.

The next paragraph describes details of the experiments conducted. For a clinical article, this could include a description of how interventions were assigned or how outcomes were measured. For a basic science article, specific details of the subsequent experiments should be provided in the order in which they were performed. Again, sufficient details should be provided so that a reader will be able to replicate the results.

Although not included in many research articles, it substantially enhances the quality of your paper if there is a paragraph discussing the sample size and power calculations used to determine the number of subjects or animals used in the study. These details help the reader understand whether the number of individuals or animals examined was sufficient to produce robust and accurate results.

The final paragraph of the Methods section usually describes the statistical analyses. In this section, report details about the different statistical tests. Explicitly state which were primary analyses and which were secondary. In addition, describe any sensitivity or subgroup analyses that were conducted; the description should indicate if these were pre-specified or post-hoc analyses. Some researchers provide information about the software used to perform the analyses. If unusual statistical tests or methodologies were used, these should be described in some detail in this section.

Results

The Results section should give the results of each of the experiments or analyses in the order they were performed. There should be a separate paragraph for each of the important experiments or analyses performed. The first paragraph is often a description of the study population. For example, the first paragraph might detail the number of patients examined, their average age, sex distribution, distribution of co-morbidities, etc. If two different groups were studied (e.g., treatment and control groups), these details should be provided in a table in two different columns.

The second paragraph goes beyond these descriptive characteristics and presents analyses that are more general. Each paragraph should address a separate topic. Avoiding all interpretation of the data in the Results section is a common mistake.

Some interpretation is permissible in this section. If you defer all discussion of the results until the Discussion section, you will have to repeat the results to contextualize the discussion for your reader. Thus, at the end of each paragraph in the Results section, a limited amount of summary and interpretation is reasonable.

Discussion

The Discussion section is the lower part of the hourglass. The beginning of the discussion is highly focused and the end is broad. I often use certain stock phrases in my first draft. In the first paragraph, I use the following: "This study was designed to..."; "We found that..."; "These results suggest that...." These sentences help formulate the first draft of my discussion. They broaden out from the narrowly focused answer to the research question and help me to apply the results in the context of the bigger picture. The second paragraph often begins, "Previous studies have found that..." and is followed by a discussion of previously published literature in this area. Place your results in the context of the existing literature, highlighting what your study adds to the literature. If your results diverge from those of previous studies, discuss the potential sources of this heterogeneity. This paragraph may be followed by additional paragraphs that are particular to the topic under discussion. Following this section, include a Limitations section.

Limitations

A discussion of the limitations of your study usually follows the Discussion section. My Limitations section often begins with: "Our study had several potential limitations...." This sentence is followed by a list of the limitations structured in the following manner: "First, ...; Second, ...; Third, ...; Finally, ..." Always present the major potential limitations of the study. However, also present the reasons that the limitation does not affect the conclusions presented in your paper. Thus, this section presents a balanced view of the strengths and weaknesses of the paper. In my papers, this section is usually one paragraph and no more than three quarters of a page in length.

Conclusions

The final paragraph of the paper is the Conclusions section. I usually structure the opening of this section in the same manner as the opening of the discussion, using the following sentences: "In conclusion, our study was designed to..."; "We found that..."; "These results suggest that...." I then include one or two additional sentences of detail. The final sentence of the paper is a major encapsulation of the message I want the reader to take from the paper. It should not be a call for further research in the area or a statement about the importance of the area. Rather, it sums up the major results and conclusions. It should allow a reader to walk away from the paper saying, "This paper is about X, and the major results were Y and Z."

References

Individual journals have specific formatting requirements for references. Check the instructions for authors for each journal prior to submission. For original research articles in general medical journals, there are usually no more than 30 references allowed. For review articles, more references can be included, perhaps 50–100. For original research articles involving many papers, such as meta-analyses, some references may be included in an appendix. Strive for the References section to include only those papers that are critical to the understanding of your paper. In general, try to have references that come from high-impact journals. Reference a limited number of review articles. Instead, the bulk of the articles should be recent original research articles. An experienced reviewer will look through the References section and note if there are no recent references present. This will signal to the reviewer that your literature search is not up-to-date.

Tables

Every paper should have some tables and/or figures. It is difficult for a reader to plow through an article that has no tables or figures to break up and clarify the text. Tables and figures help draw the reader to the important points of the paper. Limitations on the number of tables and figures are usually found in the instructions to authors issued by each journal. For an original research article, expect to see one or two tables and one or two figures, with a typical maximum of seven total tables and figures. This number can vary, however, from article to article and from journal to journal.

Examine tables from high-impact journals before putting together your own. A very simple, attractive format, such as that used by the *New England Journal of Medicine*, could be used for your initial submission. Most journals will limit the size of the tables that can be published. In general, try to limit the size of the tables so that they fit on one page of the manuscript. Tables can be presented in either letter or landscape format. Most journals ask that tables be double-spaced. However, I often use 1.0 or 1.5 spacing to fit each table on a single page.

Limit the amount of data presented in the tables. If tables are too busy, the reader will not be able to wade through all the information presented. Present only the information that is necessary to clarify and elaborate on important points. Data should be presented in either the tables or the text, not in both. If you duplicate information in this way, the journal editor will usually ask you to remove the data from one place or the other.

Table titles should be self-explanatory. If possible, avoid abbreviations in the title. Also avoid overly simplistic titles like "Clinical Characteristics". Instead, use something like "Clinical characteristics of 782 patients randomized to drug-eluting stents vs. bare metal stents". Tables are often reproduced in presentations at meetings and the title should be self-explanatory.

Take advantage of the ability to have footnotes below the table to help explain the findings. Abbreviations should be explained at the bottom of the table. Additional details that cannot be included in the table can be explained in the footnotes. For example, if 17 patients with missing data were excluded from a given analysis, this should be stated in a footnote. Examine tables from well-respected journals to get an idea of the types of information that are included in footnotes.

Figures

Each table and figure should appear on a separate page. Figures do not have their titles listed on the same page. Instead, the first figure should be labeled just "Figure 1". Provide a separate figure legend page before the tables. This page should have "Figure 1" followed by the full title of that figure and so on. Much of the information discussed regarding footnotes for tables is also applicable to figure legends. Also, in the figure legend, there is some room for interpretation of the results displayed in the figures. For example, if the graph shows a linear association between age and weight, state this below the title of the figure. This provides an opportunity to highlight the important results of the paper.

Summary

In this chapter, I have presented some tips I learned from biomedical writing courses and from my own experiences writing original research articles. Writing an original research article is one of the most important skills a physician-scientist has to learn. Helpful techniques can be learned in a biomedical writing course or by reading a book on biomedical writing. The process can also be made easier by emulating some of the stylistic methods used by experienced writers. Many writers have developed their own systematic approach, which helps them when writing their papers. It is difficult to write your first few papers. Once you have written the first few, it becomes much easier. Writing original research articles is an essential creative skill that you need to master to be a successful physician-scientist.

Key Points

- Improve your biomedical writing skills to increase your chances of publishing articles and obtaining funding for grant proposals.
- Take a formal biomedical writing course to develop your skills.

- Ask peers to critique your work.
- Use an outline to help organize your thoughts before writing a first draft.
- Try dictating your first draft.
- Use the same format each time, unless otherwise directed by a journal.
- Avoid synonyms, use short sentences and paragraphs, and use parallel structure.
- Use tables and figures to illuminate important points.
- Follow formatting/structural guidelines of the journal to which you are submitting.
- Follow an "hourglass" shape when constructing your article.

Suggested Reading

1. Cameron C, Deming SP, Notzon B, Cantor SB, Broglio KR, Pagel W. Scientific writing training for academic physicians of diverse language backgrounds. Acad Med 2009; 84: 505–510.
2. Cash TF. Caveats in the proficient preparation of an APA-style research manuscript for publication. Body Image 2009; 6: 1–6.
3. Coleman R. Tips to improve your manuscript and make the editor happy. Acta Histochem 2007; 109: 343–346.
4. Johnson TM. Tips on how to write a paper. J Am Acad Dermatol 2008; 59: 1064–1069.
5. Lee SS. How to write a paper: an editor's tips. Liver Int 2008; 28: 421–422.
6. Lin AE. Writing for scientific publication: tips for getting started. Clin Pediatr (Phila) 2006; 45: 295–300.
7. Pierson DJ. The top 10 reasons why manuscripts are not accepted for publication. Respir Care 2004; 49: 1246–1252.
8. Strunk W Jr, White EB. The Elements of Style. 4th ed. New York, NY: Longman; 1999.
9. Urrutia R. Academic skills: a concise guide to grant writing. Pancreatology 2007; 7: 307–310.
10. Zeiger M. Essentials of Writing Biomedical Research Papers. 2nd ed. San Francisco, CA: McGraw-Hill; 2000.

Chapter 10
Publishing

Productivity is never an accident. It is always the result of commitment to excellence, intelligent planning, and focused effort.

–Paul J. Myers

Introduction

In this chapter, I discuss issues related to publishing. Not only is it important to have excellent biomedical writing skills, you also need to ensure that you have a continuous stream of publications coming out of your laboratory. You need to be strategic about identifying topics for your papers and about selecting journals to send them to. As a physician-scientist, it is critical that you publish. Along with adequate grant support, publishing in high-quality journals is essential in this profession. With a strong track record, you have a greater ability to obtain grants, decline administrative responsibilities, and advance academically; in short, you will be more independent if you have a solid stream of publications.

Why Produce a Continuous Stream of Publications?

It is essential to produce a constant stream of publications during your career. You need to demonstrate continuous productivity to maintain your protected time for research. If your research productivity tapers off, those in charge of scheduling will see little reason to provide you with protected time. In order to increase or even maintain your protected time, you need to demonstrate a continuous stream of high-quality publications. You also need to demonstrate a continuous stream of high-quality publications for promotion purposes and to enhance your ability to obtain grants. If there is a gap of one or more years between first and senior author publications, it will be viewed unfavorably by promotion and grant review committees. You also need to demonstrate continued productivity to obtain career awards. If you cannot demonstrate continuous productivity in terms of first and senior author publications, it will be difficult to obtain this type of support. Similarly, if you have a gap of one or two years without salary support, your protected time may decrease, as will your ability to generate research.

Always plan the next few years of your career strategically. Conduct multiple on-going projects. Some of these projects will be short-term, some medium-term, and some long-term. A continuous pipeline of projects and manuscripts will ensure that you are able to produce a continuous stream of high-quality publications. This stream should include one or two first-author publications per year, with at least several other publications as senior author. The ratio between first and senior author publications changes as you become more senior. In the early stages of your career, a greater proportion of your publications will be as first author; whereas, at later stages, you will have more as senior author. Although it is useful and expected that you be a middle author on some multi-author publications, these types of publications should not be at the expense of your first and senior author publications.

Types of Projects to Tackle

You are a new assistant professor with start up funds and protected time for research. You believe that now is the time to undertake an ambitious long-term project that you have not been able to take on earlier in your career. Although I agree that you can and should begin more ambitious projects, do not take on projects that are too long in scope and that are perhaps not feasible to accomplish as an assistant professor. As a new assistant professor, you typically have three–five years to demonstrate research productivity. In many institutions, if you have not obtained an operating grant, produced some high-quality first-author publications, and perhaps obtained a career award during this time, you might be obligated to go to full-time clinician status.

Therefore, during the first few years, it is crucial that you establish a solid research team and a pipeline of projects to ensure that you are continually producing publications. Since three–five years is a short timeline, be circumspect in your selection of projects. Although you may choose to focus some of your energy on projects with a greater timeline, plan the bulk of your projects so that papers will be published within five years of the start of your appointment as an assistant professor. Therefore, it is helpful to begin several small original research projects that are more likely to produce results within one–two years. You can spearhead some of these projects, while medical students, residents, fellows, or graduate students under your supervision can spearhead others. Most research projects take much more time than initially anticipated. Thus, you have to be modest in your expectations at the beginning of your career.

To bolster your publication record and have a continuous pipeline of publications, consider writing some articles that do not involve original research, such as narrative reviews, systematic reviews, meta-analyses, book chapters, research letters, and editorials (Table 10.1). In general, systematic reviews and meta-analyses

Table 10.1 Types of biomedical publications

Type of publication	Definition
Abstract	Brief summary of original research study, usually no more than 250 words
Book	Academic or otherwise, of which you are the primary author or editor
Book chapter	Contribution to a book of which you are not the primary author
Consensus statement	Consensus about an issue by a group of experts which is used to guide policy
Editorial	Comments on previous article or opinions on a topic (usually by a senior investigator and usually invited)
Guideline statement	Comprehensive review of literature by a group of experts with recommendations for practice
Lay press	Article in non-scientific journal for the dissemination of information to the general public
Meta-analysis	Statistical summary of findings from original research articles identified in a systematic literature search
Narrative review	Qualitative review combining primary studies, theories, and author experience
Original research article	Report, interpretation, and discussion of original research
Research letter (RL)/Brief report (BR)	Similar to original research article but typically no more than 600 (RL) or 1,500 (BR) words
Systematic review	Literature review that systematically synthesizes and discusses all high-quality research relevant to a question

are the most highly regarded of these. Do not spend too much time on book reviews or editorials, and compose a research letter only when you do not have enough material for a full manuscript. Nevertheless, a mix of such publications can add a lot to your publication record. It is ideal to always have one or two of these articles on the go, in addition to your original research projects. Although these types of articles are not as highly regarded by promotions committees, it is helpful to publish several of these papers during the first few years of your career. These articles should not make up the bulk of your CV, but they will help establish you as an authority in your area, give you credibility as first or senior author, and they can serve as the background section of a grant application or a protocol for a research project.

You are often in an excellent position to identify possible topics for these types of articles. Because of your clinical activities, you are in close touch with at least one specific area of medical practice. Within this area, there are many "hot" topics with unanswered questions. Clinicians appreciate guidance for contentious clinical issues. New diagnostic techniques, treatments, and devices may have been evaluated in a number of small studies; however, the results of these studies may not have been pooled. A systematic review of the available data might be extremely helpful to clinicians in making informed decisions about which techniques, treatments, and devices to incorporate into their practice.

Narrative Reviews

Narrative reviews do not involve systematic pooling of data. Instead, previous studies are summarized and discussed. This type of review provides clinicians with a more comprehensive understanding of the current literature on a given topic. Narrative reviews may be biased, however. The authors of narrative reviews can be selective in their inclusion of publications. If they have a particular bias for or against a technique or therapy, authors can select the articles they present and sway clinicians depending on how they present the evidence. Despite this, narrative reviews can still be useful. For example, if a topic is too vast to allow a comprehensive systematic review, a narrative review is an effective way of summarizing and comparing the most recent or relevant data. However, when feasible, a systematic review is preferable.

Systematic Reviews

Like narrative reviews, systematic reviews focus on a particular subject but do not statistically pool the results of the studies. Instead, a systematic review typically provides a paragraph reviewing each of the relevant studies. The main result of a systematic review might be a table or a series of tables in which the results of the original research investigations of a particular topic are clearly laid out.

Systematic reviews are very useful for clinicians because they review the entire literature on a particular topic in a systematic and unbiased way. Tables or figures in which the original research on a particular topic is summarized allow a clinician to quickly decide whether a particular technique, therapy, or diagnostic test is useful or not.

Unlike narrative reviews, systematic reviews employ an organized and comprehensive approach to obtaining and evaluating the literature. Specific criteria are used to conduct and report systematic reviews. Study the methodology for a systematic review before embarking upon a project of this kind. Systematic review methodology helps you avoid biases when summarizing the literature. Using predetermined inclusion/exclusion criteria, a systematic review limits the possibility for bias compared to traditional narrative reviews. Many systematic reviews also employ scoring systems to evaluate the quality of the papers that are included in the review.

Systematic reviews should not be large-scope articles that cover an entire syndrome or disease. Instead, they should focus on a narrow topic and review the relevant randomized controlled trials (RCTs) and observational studies. Systematic reviews should have a limited and clearly stated number of objectives. At the end of your systematic review, provide the clinician with specific recommendations about the use of a particular technique or procedure, or diagnostic test. Ask yourself the following types of questions: is it worthwhile? Is it worthwhile only in certain subgroups of patients? Are there questions that need to be answered before it can be used extensively? Is it safe? Is there enough data to give a definitive answer? If this is not yet the case, what studies are needed for a definitive answer? These are the types of issues that clinicians want to know about and that will improve the likelihood of your article being published in a high-impact journal.

Besides providing additional publications while you are working on your original research projects, systematic reviews can complement the original research projects being conducted in your laboratory. For example, whenever you write a grant proposal, the background section needs to include a systematic review of the current literature. Many systematic reviews are background sections from grants, which the author has expanded and published. Create the maximum number of publications from the work you are conducting. If you have written an excellent grant proposal, why not use the background section and publish it as a systematic review? This may require an extra 20% effort, but it will result in an additional publication and will be well worth the effort.

Meta-analyses

In a meta-analysis, data from relevant articles are synthesized. By statistically analyzing and comparing data across RCTs, an investigator can draw conclusions based on a larger sample size than that of each individual RCT. Meta-analyses are a hybrid-type of article because they produce original conclusions from non-original data.

Some scientists consider them to be original research articles, while others consider them to be systematic review articles. Conducting a meta-analysis is a very beneficial endeavor for a new physician-scientist. Since these articles involve pooling data that have already been reported in the literature, they can be put together relatively quickly. In addition, strong meta-analyses are often published in high-impact journals. The sample size of a meta-analysis is much greater than that of any individual study because many studies are pooled. For this reason, results from meta-analyses are often of great interest to practicing clinicians. Because of this, it is often possible to obtain grant support for meta-analyses from funding agencies. This is useful with respect to conducting the research, and it will add to your credentials.

Specific guidelines govern the design and reporting of meta-analyses. If you have no training in epidemiology or biostatistics, include an experienced clinical epidemiologist in your research team. Read the literature on how to perform and report a meta-analysis. Various measures can be used to assess the quality of the studies you include in your meta-analysis (e.g., Jadad scores), while the PRISMA statement provides authoritative guidance on how to perform and report meta-analyses.

It is important to assess all available studies to make sure it is possible to include them in a meta-analysis. To begin with, the topic should have at least five studies that can be pooled. Pooling fewer than five studies is not likely to produce worthwhile results. In addition, the studies need to define variables in a similar way and report data using similar measures for the studies to be comparable. If there are insufficient studies or if they are not sufficiently similar for statistical pooling, it is likely better to conduct a systematic review.

It is advantageous to conduct a meta-analysis while pursuing your primary research projects. Make sure you have multiple projects in various stages of completion and multiple articles in various stages of preparation, so that you can maintain a constant flow in your pipeline of publications. You need to demonstrate productivity within the first few years of your career. Collecting original data is often time-consuming. If you exclusively choose projects involving original data collection, you may have little to show after your first few years. For this reason, consider performing one or more meta-analyses at the beginning of your career. Well-written meta-analyses can result in high-impact publications that are completed more quickly than your original research publications. Meta-analyses often have a major impact on clinical practice.

Editorials

It is unlikely that you will be invited to write editorials at an early stage of your career. These invitations occur more frequently when you are a more senior investigator. However, high-impact journals do publish the occasional unsolicited editorial from a young investigator. This may occur when a young investigator submits an uninvited review article. If the article deals with a controversial topic, the editors will sometimes choose to publish the revised article as an editorial. Occasionally, you may be successful in submitting an uninvited editorial if you have a particular viewpoint on a contentious contemporary issue.

Book Chapters and Books

Book chapters are much less highly valued by promotions and grant review committees than peer-reviewed original research articles. You likely will be asked to write some book chapters at the beginning of your career. Limit your time in this regard. While it is beneficial to publish the occasional book chapter, it is best to reserve the bulk of your time for articles that will be published in the peer-reviewed medical literature. Particularly at the beginning of your career, you may be invited to write a book chapter as a co-author with a more senior author. Although you will be the first author, the senior author will be recognized as the established physician-scientist. As a result, promotions and grant review committees do not usually value book chapters very highly; they put more stock in articles published in the peer-reviewed medical literature.

It is also possible that you will be approached to write a book early in your career. Although this is unusual, it does happen. Again, be circumspect in your decision to accept this kind of time commitment. Writing a book requires large amounts of time, which will detract from your original research activities. At the beginning of your career, establish your research team, obtain funding, and ensure a continuous pipeline of projects and publications. Because your time is limited, do not invest it in writing a book at this stage of your career. Consider writing a book once you become a more established investigator (ideally with tenure).

Choosing a Topic

I consider several factors when deciding on a topic for an article that does not involve original research. First, is the subject topical? If the subject has been reviewed many times in the past and is not currently an active issue, I do not consider it. To have a paper published in a high-impact journal, you need to write about a topic that is of current clinical interest and that may even be contentious. Perform a PubMed search to see if any recent reviews have been published in high-impact journals. If articles have been published only in moderate or low-impact journals, it may still be worthwhile to proceed. It is important to note that from the time you first begin to write your article, it will take at least a year to get it published. As a result, even if a review article on your topic was published a year ago, by the time your article is published, it will be two years since the topic was last reviewed. However, if there are multiple recent review articles on this subject in high-impact journals, choose another topic. You do not want to spend considerable time on an article addressing a topic that will be over-reviewed by the time you are ready to publish.

A second consideration is whether there have been enough published articles on this topic for you to systematically collect them and synthesize them. If you want to review a particular diagnostic test or therapy, you should do a PubMed search to see if a sufficient number of original research articles have been published on this topic. If fewer than five original research articles have been published, there may not be enough evidence for you to put together a worthwhile review. On the other hand, if you find more than 100 articles on this topic, choose another subject. The subject area is too large, and there is no way that you can do it justice in a review article. One way to approach this issue is to see whether there is one aspect of the topic that you could investigate. For example, I had a fellow who really wanted to write a review article on IIb/IIIa inhibitors. I knew that this topic was problematic because there were hundreds of studies already published, as well as many review articles. Instead, I had him focus on IIb/IIIa inhibitors in the setting of treatment for acute myocardial infarction. This was a more manageable topic.

This brings up a third consideration. Your topic should be as focused as possible. The more focused your topic, the more meaningful your synthesis of the literature and the more specific your recommendations. Also, the more focused your topic is, the fewer articles you will have to deal with. You can analyze these articles in much greater depth than you can in a review article that covers a much larger scope.

Finally, editors of high-impact journals are often interested in publishing uninvited review articles on topics of compelling interest. These topics include new therapeutic modalities, new diagnostic modalities, new classes of medications, or new procedures. Editors are typically not interested in review articles on topics that have been reviewed extensively in the literature. Therefore, review articles on clinical syndromes that have been well-recognized for many years are not usually of interest, unless there have been recent findings that change our understanding of the syndrome. Carefully consider how innovative and compelling your question or approach is when choosing a topic.

There are many ways to identify questions you might want to address in your research. Think about the questions that come up in the course of your clinical activities. Query your clinical colleagues about the types of topics they think would be particularly relevant and compelling. When I attend national and international meetings, I often jot down ideas for topics while I am listening to various presentations. I always maintain a list of 5–10 topics for potential articles. Medical students, residents, fellows, and graduate students often contact me about possible research topics. In addition to giving them an original research project, I often give them a review article to write at the same time. This gives them the opportunity to get their hands wet writing while they are collecting data for their project. If you keep your eyes and ears open for research questions during your clinical activities, you will always have a substantial list of ideas from which to choose a new project. From this list, choose the ones that have not already been addressed extensively in other publications, that have enough studies available to conduct a worthwhile review, that can be focused to provide specific, useful recommendations, and that are extremely compelling topics.

Choosing a Journal

Choosing a journal for your manuscript can be a difficult task. New physician-scientists often make the mistake of submitting their articles to journals that are too low in caliber. The caliber of a journal is often assessed by its impact factor, which indicates the frequency with which articles from a given journal are cited. A given journal's impact factor is calculated by dividing the number of current-year citations of articles published in that journal by the number of articles published in the journal over the previous two years (Tables 10.2). Journal impact factors are accessible on the web. Publishing your article in a high-impact journal is more advantageous to your career than publishing it in a low-impact journal. Why not start with a high-impact journal, even though it may not be accepted? Although your chances of being published in a high-impact journal may be small, there is no harm in submitting your manuscripts to these journals and it is often worthwhile. There is one reason for this; it may be accepted! If so, it would be a shame to have published in a low-impact journal instead.

It generally takes several months for a journal to review your article. Even if your article is rejected, you will receive reviews of your article from knowledgeable reviewers who are often authorities in your subject area. Based on their reviews, you may choose to revise your article before submitting to the next journal on your list. This is not my practice, however. If one of my articles is rejected from a high-impact journal, I usually submit it immediately to the next journal lower down on the impact factor list without revising it. I revise articles only when a journal has indicated that it may be interested in publishing it. This is important, because if you decide that you are going to revise your article before submitting to the next journal, it may be several months before you submit it. Rather than losing time, submit your article to the next journal on your list as soon as you get a rejection. You know which journals in your area are high-impact. Start with the highest and move down the list. Remember, there is always a journal that will publish your article. Even when an article has been rejected by many journals, keep on submitting it until it gets published. You have gone to all the work of writing a manuscript, so it is worthwhile putting in the effort to get it published. This is true even if it is published in a journal that is not indexed in PubMed.

Revisions

Once a journal indicates interest in publishing your article, they usually require revisions. Several months after you first submit your manuscript, the response comes back from the journal's editors. They may say that they are interested in publishing your manuscript pending revisions. This means that they are not committing to publishing your manuscript but are likely to publish it if you adequately address the comments from their reviewers. Sometimes, their responses are so non-committal, you may think that they have rejected your article. This is not the case. They just

Table 10.2 Impact factor 2008: top 10

Rank	Journal title	Total cites	Articles	Impact factor (IF)
General and Internal Medicine				
1	*New England Journal of Medicine*	205, 750	356	50.0
2	*Journal of the American Medical Association*	114, 250	225	31.7
3	*Lancet*	148, 106	289	28.4
4	*Annals of Internal Medicine*	44, 785	162	17.5
5	*British Medical Journal*	68, 464	281	12.8
6	*Public Library of Science Medicine*	6, 075	133	12.2
7	*Annual Review of Medicine*	4, 057	34	11.0
8	*Archives of Internal Medicine*	35, 176	262	9.1
9	*Canadian Medical Association Journal*	9, 606	105	7.5
10	*Annals of Medicine*	3, 222	64	5.4
Research and Experimental Medicine				
1	*Nature Medicine*	48, 632	143	27.6
2	*Journal of Clinical Investigation*	87, 012	353	16.6
3	*Journal of Experimental Medicine*	67, 322	245	15.2
4	*Trends in Molecular Medicine*	4, 280	60	9.6
5	*Molecular Aspects of Medicine*	1, 513	35	7.3
6	*Molecular Therapy*	8, 301	234	6.0
7	*Current Molecular Medicine*	2, 159	72	5.3
8	*Journal of Cellular and Molecular Medicine*	2, 432	226	5.1
9	*Laboratory Investigation*	10, 225	117	4.6
10	*Gene Therapy*	9, 157	173	4.5
Cardiac and Cardiovascular Systems				
1	*Circulation*	143, 852	607	14.6
2	*Journal of the American College of Cardiology*	60, 121	462	11.4
3	*Circulation Research*	39, 873	320	10.0
4	*European Heart Journal*	21, 703	296	8.9
5	*Nature Clinical Practice Cardiovascular Medicine*	978	81	6.0
6	*Cardiovascular Research*	16, 079	272	5.9
7	*Basic Research in Cardiology*	2, 266	57	5.4
8	*Journal of Molecular and Cellular Cardiology*	9, 279	179	5.1
9	*Heart*	11, 162	232	5.0
10	*Progress in Cardiovascular Diseases*	1, 716	34	4.7
Multidisciplinary Sciences				
1	*Nature*	443, 967	899	31.4
2	*Science*	409, 290	862	28.1
3	*Proceedings of the National Academy of Sciences*	416, 018	3508	9.4
4	*Nano Today*	376	13	8.8
5	*IBM Journal of Research and Development*	3, 547	51	3.7
6	*Journal of the Royal Society Interface*	1, 111	154	3.6
7	*Scientific American*	5, 317	88	2.3
8	*Annals of the New York Academy of Sciences*	37, 539	975	2.3
9	*Philosophical Transactions of the Royal Society A*	8, 012	276	2.3
10	*Naturwissenschaften*	4, 692	154	2.1

1. ISI Web of Knowledge 2008 Journal Citation Reports. http://admin-apps.isiknowledge.com/JCR/JCR. Accessed August 4, 2009.

want to make sure that they have the opportunity to reject your article if they do not think that your revisions are adequate. If they indicate that they are potentially interested, revise the manuscript, respond to the reviewers' comments, and resubmit. You have two tasks: (1) prepare a letter of response addressing the reviewers' comments; and (2) revise the article. For most journals, you will receive comments from two or more reviewers. The manuscript is sent to these external reviewers. They read the manuscript and send back their comments and their recommendations about whether your article should be published. Depending on the journal and the topic of your paper, there may be a statistical reviewer as well. Usually, the editors also provide comments.

It is important to spend time composing a letter of response to the reviewers' comments. This letter is extremely important, and it often makes the difference to your article being accepted for publication or not. In this letter, respond to the reviewers' comments in the order they appear and in detail. Starting with reviewer 1, list in bold or italics the verbatim comment from the reviewer. Next, provide a short paragraph indicating whether you agree with the comment or not. You may agree with the reviewer's comment and indicate the page and paragraph where you made the suggested changes. Alternately, you may state that you do not agree with the reviewer and explain why.

It is important that you systematically address each of the reviewers' comments in the order in which they are presented. It is also essential to list each of the comments verbatim as you prepare the letter of response. The editors will review your letter to ensure that you addressed each of the comments. They want to see that you have taken the comments seriously. You do not need to revise your article in response to each of the comments. However, you do need to give a considered response to each comment. Be diplomatic when composing this letter, even when the reviewers are not! Close with a sentences such as the following: "We thank the reviewers and the editors for their comments. We have revised the article with respect to their comments and we think that it has been significantly improved. Thank you for your help. We look forward to your response."

In addition to responding to reviewers' comments, you need to revise the manuscript itself. In some cases, the revisions are minor; in other cases, the revisions are major. If you state that you revised a section of the manuscript in your letter of response, make sure that you do. Revising often takes the form of giving more detail about a particular issue. For example, a reviewer may say that you did not discuss a potential bias in your limitations section. In that case, mention in your letter that you agree with the reviewer and have addressed the issue in the limitations section of your paper on page X. In your article, include a short paragraph about the potential bias and why you do not think that it affects the conclusions of your paper.

In some cases, reviewers will ask for additional analyses or experiments. As much as possible, try to perform these analyses or experiments. If they are not feasible, say so and explain why. Similarly, if a limitation is insurmountable due to the nature of the data or for some other reason, mention this and make a case for why your study is the best possible way to answer the question. It is always worthwhile to resubmit the paper to the journal, even if you are not able to perform all the analyses or experiments or implement all the suggested changes. Just address the comments and explain why they are beyond the scope of this paper or why they are not feasible.

If the editor suggests that certain changes are mandatory, I would definitely do them. For example, if they ask you to shorten the text, you clearly need to do this. If they ask you to remove a table, you need to do it. The editors are the ones who decide whether or not your paper will be published. If they ask you to do something, make sure to comply with their requests. Occasionally, in your letter of response, you can say that you think that the paper is much stronger with the inclusion of the table, but that you are willing to defer to the editors on this issue.

Once you submit your letter of response and your revised manuscript, you will again have to wait weeks before getting a response. The wait may sometimes be as long as it took to review your paper in the first place. The editors usually make the final decision on their own. Occasionally, they will send your revised manuscript and letter of response back to the reviewers for their opinions. Hopefully, at the end of this time, the article will be accepted. Occasionally, additional minor revisions will be requested. Finally, some journals have you go through the entire revision process and ultimately decide to decline your manuscript. There is not much you can do if this occurs; just start over again and submit to the next journal on your list.

There is an appeal process at journals to which you can turn if you feel that you have been dealt with unfairly. In my experience, however, this process usually does not reverse the decision, and it often wastes your time for several more months. It is unfortunate that some editors state that they will potentially accept your article pending major revisions and then ultimately reject it. However, you usually do not have much recourse in this situation. Just turn around and submit to the next journal.

Summary

One of the keys to having a successful research career is to have a continuous pipeline of publications. You need to have a variety of short-term, medium-term, and ambitious long-term projects in the works. There needs to be a continuous stream of publications from your laboratory. This stream can include a mix of original research articles, narrative reviews, systematic reviews, meta-analyses, book chapters, research letters, and editorials. Needless to say, the greatest percentage of your publications should be original research articles. Make sure that you regularly publish articles on which you are the first or senior author. It is not auspicious for your career if most of your publications are multi-author and you are one of the middle authors. The key to having a continuous stream of publications is perseverance. Often, a paper is rejected by journal after journal. Do not give up hope. There is always a journal that will ultimately publish your article. Even if it has been rejected by multiple journals, keep on resubmitting until you find a journal that is willing to publish it. It is a shame to go to all the work of writing a paper and not have it published. As you progress in your career, you will become much more adept at the ins and outs of publishing. Writing articles will become easier; maintaining a pipeline of projects will become easier; and dealing with journals and rejections will become easier. No matter where you are in your career, the process of transforming one of your ideas into a project, following it through to data collection, data analysis, manuscript writing, and ultimately publication will still give you great satisfaction.

Key Points

- Maintain a steady output of high-quality publications to maintain protected time and salary support and to obtain promotions and peer-reviewed funding.
- Have multiple projects on the burner simultaneously; short, medium, and long term.
- At the beginning of your career, select projects that you can complete and publish in three–five years.
- Write occasional review articles, meta-analyses, book chapters, research letters, and editorials.
- Examine questions that arise in your clinical practice.
- Submit to the highest impact journal, then the next highest, and so on.
- If asked, revise your article and prepare a letter of response.
- Respond to each of the reviewers' comments and explain why you did or did not make the proposed change.
- Most of your publications should be first or senior author original research articles.

Suggested Reading

1. Altman DG, Schulz KF, Moher D, et al. The revised CONSORT statement for reporting randomized trials: explanation and elaboration. Ann Intern Med 2001; 134: 663–694.
2. Bordage G. Reasons reviewers reject and accept manuscripts: the strengths and weaknesses in medical education reports. Acad Med 2001; 76: 889–896.
3. Bourne PE. Ten simple rules for getting published. PLoS Comput Biol 2005; 1: e57.
4. DeBehnke DJ, Kline JA, Shih RD. Research fundamentals: choosing an appropriate journal, manuscript preparation, and interactions with editors. Acad Emerg Med 2001; 8: 844–850.
5. Liberati A, Altman DG, Tetzlaff J, et al. The PRISMA statement for reporting systematic reviews and meta-analyses of studies that evaluate health care interventions: explanation and elaboration. PLoS Med 2009; 6: e1000100.
6. Lopez-Abente G, Munoz-Tinoco C. Time trends in the impact factor of Public Health journals. BMC Public Health 2005; 5: 24.
7. Moher D, Liberati A, Tetzlaff J, Altman DG. Preferred reporting items for systematic reviews and meta-analyses: the PRISMA statement. PLoS Med 2009; 6: e1000097.
8. Overcash JA. Narrative research: a review of methodology and relevance to clinical practice. Crit Rev Oncol Hematol 2003; 48: 179–184.
9. Rau JL. Searching the literature and selecting the right references. Respir Care 2004; 49: 1242–1245.

10. Samet JM. Dear author - advice from a retiring editor. Am J Epidemiol 1999; 150: 433–436.
11. Sayers A. Tips and tricks in performing a systematic review - chapter 4. Br J Gen Pract 2008; 58: 136.
12. Thompson PJ. How to choose the right journal for your manuscript. Chest 2007; 132: 1073–1076.

Chapter 11
Grants

Money never starts an idea. It is always the idea that starts the money.

–Owen Laughlin

Introduction

Obtaining peer-reviewed grant support is one of your major goals as a new physician-scientist. Because obtaining grant support is such an important and extensive topic, I have divided my discussion into three chapters: Chapter 11, Grants; Chapter 12, Grantsmanship; and Chapter 13, Peer Review of Grant Applications. This chapter deals with the following issues:

- What are grants and why are they important?
- Where do you apply for grants?
- What types of grants are available?
- How does an operating grant differ from a career award?

The chapter on Grantsmanship deals with these issues:

- What strategic issues should you be aware of when deciding on a topic?
- How do you choose the right funding agency and committee?
- How do you structure your grant and optimize your chances of obtaining funding?

The chapter on Peer Review of Grant Applications is my account of one of the grant review committee meetings I attended and the tips I learned. Having an insider's knowledge of what goes on in these meetings will give you greater insight into how to write grants that are more likely to be funded. Obtaining grant support is critical to your success as a physician-scientist. Having a good grasp of the essentials of the application process is important to your success. It may take several years of trial and error before you have a thorough understanding of the vocabulary

M.J. Eisenberg, *The Physician Scientist's Career Guide,*
DOI 10.1007/978-1-60327-908-6_11, © Springer Science+Business Media, LLC 2011

and the process associated with the grant application process. These three chapters are not an exhaustive treatment of the topic, but I hope that reading them will help increase your understanding and your ability to obtain funding.

What Are Grants and Why Are They Important?

A grant is a sum of money given to you by a funding agency to allow you to conduct research. Some grants provide money to conduct a research project (i.e., research grants or operating grants); other grants provide you with money to supplement your salary so that you have protected time to work on your research projects (i.e., career development awards or salary support grants). Because the demand for grants is much greater than the funds available, a competitive peer-review process is used to determine which applications will be funded. To apply for research funding, you must submit your application to an agency that funds research grants. In North America, most agencies currently fund less than 25% of grant applications. As a result, for you to be successful in obtaining grants, you need a thorough understanding of what grants are available, where to apply for them, and how to put together a strong application.

Obtaining grant support is important for two reasons. First, you need funding to conduct your research projects. Without funding, you cannot hire laboratory personnel or purchase the equipment and materials required for your research. As a junior physician-scientist, you might not require large amounts of funding. As you become more senior, however, your projects may become more ambitious in scope and require more extensive funding. At any stage of your career, the ability to attract peer-reviewed funding is critical for you to be able to conduct your research.

A second reason for obtaining grant support is that it is one of the central issues examined when you are being considered for promotion. You need to demonstrate the ability to obtain peer-reviewed grant support in order to be promoted from assistant to associate professor and from associate to full professor. Success at obtaining peer-reviewed grant support is also essential to obtaining tenure. As a result, a solid understanding of the types of grants available and how to obtain them is an important part of your knowledge base as a physician-scientist.

The following discussion focuses on research grants available in the United States and Canada. Nevertheless, much of the following discussion applies to funding agencies in most countries.

Where to Apply for Grants

There are two major sources of grant support. The first, and by far the most important source, is the government. The second is non-governmental organizations including foundations, industry, and professional associations. Government sources include federal, state, or provincial agencies, and occasionally local agencies. In most countries including the United States and Canada, the majority of research grants are funded by federal agencies. In the United States and Canada, the major funding agencies are the National Institutes of Health (NIH) and the Canadian Institutes for Health Research (CIHR), respectively. Obtaining funding from a federal agency is considered a high achievement.

In both the United States and Canada, many state and provincial funding agencies also provide grant support. The type of research supported, the budgets available, and the duration of the grants provided vary from agency to agency. Typically, budgets supplied by state or provincial agencies are less than those provided by federal agencies. In addition, some state and provincial agencies prefer to fund new investigators, because they often have a hard time competing for peer-reviewed support at the federal level. By focusing on new investigators, these agencies help them become established so that they will have a better chance of obtaining federal grant support in the future. Some local agencies also support biomedical research. In general, however, budgets for these agencies are usually small, and the specifics of the grants they fund also vary substantially among different localities.

Federal Sources of Funding

National Institutes of Health (NIH)

The NIH is the major peer-reviewed funding agency of the United States' federal government. The NIH provides the majority of the funding available to American researchers. It is a huge bureaucracy with multiple institutes and centers. In 2010, it consisted of 20 institutes and 7 centers. Each agency has its own mission statement and as a result, its own particular priorities with respect to research. You should be aware of these priorities when you submit your application. If you can frame your research project so that it falls within the domain of one or more of the NIH institutes or centers, your chances of obtaining funding will be enhanced. Importantly, the NIH is one of the few funding agencies in the world that will fund outside investigators. If you are applying for NIH funding and do not reside in the United States, you normally have to show that the research cannot be performed in the United States and that it is relevant to the citizens of the United States. However, it would still be strategic to include an American researcher as a co-investigator on your project.

Canadian Institutes of Health Research (CIHR)

The CIHR is analogous to the NIH and is Canada's federal agency responsible for funding health research in Canada. The CIHR consists of 13 institutes such as the Institute of Circulatory and Respiratory Health, the Institute of Infection and Immunity, and the Institute of Aging. Each institute has a mandate to fund grant applications within their disciplines. The institutes identify important research areas, build research capacity in under-developed areas, help train health researchers, and support knowledge translation so that research results are translated into practice.

State, Provincial, and Local Sources of Funding

State, provincial, and local sources of funding vary greatly. In the province of Quebec where I reside, for example, the agency responsible for funding health research offers operating grants only to new investigators, but it offers career awards to junior, mid- and senior-level investigators. I encourage you to explore the offerings of your regional and local sources of funding. When available, they can significantly boost your research agenda, especially as a new investigator.

Non-Governmental Sources of Funding

Non-governmental or private sources of funding can be a significant source of grant support for physician-scientists. They include foundations, industry, and professional associations.

Foundations

For many physician-scientists, foundations are a primary source of grant support. Many diseases have their own foundations to which you can apply. For example, in the United States, the American Heart Association and the National Cancer Society are two organizations that provide funding for research in cardiovascular disease and cancer, respectively. Other foundations focus on diseases like diabetes, renal failure, and rheumatoid arthritis. Canada has similar foundations. Foundations usually have specific mandates in terms of the type of research they fund. For this reason, closely examine the mission statement of each foundation before applying for grant support. Importantly, the budgets available from these foundations are typically smaller than those available from federal agencies.

Industry

Industry can also be a significant source of funding for new physician-scientists. Many pharmaceutical companies support investigator-initiated grant proposals (see Chapter 17 for more details). An effective way to find out whether a particular pharmaceutical company accepts submissions for investigator-initiated grant proposals is by speaking to the company representative who serves your hospital. This individual can put you in touch with the right people at their company. For an investigator-initiated application, a company may request a one- or two-page summary of your proposal. If they are interested in your proposal, they will request a full application. This application includes the full protocol of the study as well as a budget and budget justification. Pharmaceutical companies typically have limited scope in terms of funding grant proposals. They are often interested only in proposals that have to do with their products. You need to carefully consider this issue when you are composing an investigator-initiated grant proposal.

Similar to foundations, the amount of funding available from industry sources is usually relatively small compared to that available from federal funding agencies. For this reason, it is worthwhile to discuss this issue with them. Once you know the maximum budget and duration that they typically fund, you can identify whether the scope of your study falls within these parameters.

Professional Associations

Some professional associations provide small amounts of funding for research projects. The budgets from these associations are usually small, and these organizations often have specific mission statements, thereby limiting the types of research projects they can fund. Before applying, closely examine what they are looking for to make sure it will accommodate your interests.

Types of Operating Grants

There are many types of operating grants available. The type of research supported, the amounts awarded, the duration of the awards, and the type of researchers funded varies substantially from agency to agency. Detailing all the different types of grants that are available is well beyond the scope of this chapter. Below, however, I briefly discuss some of the major types of grants available from the NIH. I also include a list of major NIH and CIHR grants in Appendices 3 and 4, respectively. For more details about the type of grants you can apply for, consult the websites of the NIH, the CIHR, and other agencies that you are interested in.

Research Grants (R Series)

The series of research grants offered by the NIH is known as the R series. Besides the RO1 grant, this series includes the RO3 Small Grant Program, the R13 Conferences and Scientific Meetings Grant, the R34 Clinical Trial Planning Grant and others (Appendix 3).

The RO1 grant is the basic investigator-initiated grant program to which physician-scientists apply to obtain operating funds from the NIH. It is usually the first operating grant you apply for as a new physician-scientist. If you already have your own idea for a research project and want to obtain funding from the NIH, you will normally prepare an RO1 grant application.

Applications for new RO1s are accepted in February, June, and October. The earliest the awards are announced are December, April, and July, respectively. As a result, 9–10 months elapse between the time you apply and the time the funds arrive. If your grant is rejected, you have several months to revise it before submitting it to the next competition. It is important when preparing your first application that you examine the NIH website to identify when the application is due and where it should be sent. Funding agencies are very strict about their requirements regarding grant submissions. If you do not respect the agency deadlines, your application will be rejected and you will have to wait until the next competition to re-submit it.

Invited Grant Applications

In addition to the RO1 program, there are many other grant programs you can submit to. Many of these programs involve invited grant applications. The concept behind these programs is to identify areas of high importance and invite applications in these areas. The chance of being funded if you apply to one of these programs is greater than the chance of being funded if you apply through the RO1 competition. Fewer than 25% of unsolicited RO1 applications are funded. As a result, you need to keep informed about the individual grant programs. If you can frame your research idea so that it meets their criteria, you will have a better chance of being funded than if you submit the same application to an RO1 competition.

The NIH has a language of its own that requires years to master. I list the definitions for several of the terms they use in Appendix 5. However, you particularly need to be aware of the following two acronyms: RFAs and PAs. Requests for applications (RFAs) refer to invitations from the NIH to submit applications that deal with particular research issues. Often, an RFA is issued only once. There is generally a fixed budget for the entire program, a fixed duration for the applications, as well as a maximum amount of funding that you can request. The grant department at your medical center, university, or research institute keeps track of current RFAs and will inform you as soon as they are announced. Make sure that you are on the appropriate email lists so that you are notified immediately about all announcements regarding RFAs.

Program announcements (PAs) are more general than RFAs. PAs involve requests for grant applications in a general area of major interest to the funding agency. For example, diabetes or obesity might be areas for program announcements. Similar to RFAs, PAs let you know that the funding agency is particularly interested in inviting grant applications in this area. If you submit an application in this area, you will have a greater chance of being funded than if you submit a topic in a non-priority area. As a result, try to frame your research question to fit the requirements of a PA. If you have not settled on your research program when you first start your career as a physician-scientist, it will be helpful to review the current PAs in your area of interest. Putting together a research program in an area considered important by a federal agency will make it much easier for you to get your program funded.

Experienced physician-scientists make a point of submitting grant applications in response to RFAs and PAs. If you are a new physician-scientist, you might not have this mindset. Most new physician-scientists are not aware of the importance of RFAs and PAs. They usually develop an original idea for a research project and submit their application to the general competition. However, competition among unsolicited submissions is great. As a new investigator, you are not as well equipped as a more experienced senior investigator to submit a competitive application. As a result, the likelihood of obtaining funding in an open competition may be small. It is true that both the NIH and CIHR make an effort to fund new investigators. However, your application is still in competition with those of mid-career and senior investigators. If possible, put together an application that is relevant to an RFA or a PA. Your chances of being funded will be significantly enhanced.

Letter of Intent (LOI)

Some funding agencies require an LOI in advance of inviting a full grant proposal. Although you may view this as a delay in submitting your proposal, it can save you a lot of time and heartache. Rather than preparing a full-length proposal, you can prepare a one- to two-page LOI that outlines the rationale, study design, and an abbreviated budget of your research proposal. The LOI is reviewed by the funding agency to decide whether they are interested in seeing your full proposal. If they are, they will request a complete grant application from you. If they are not, they will tell you so. This process can save you time and effort by letting you know in advance whether your topic is of interest before you go through the lengthy process of preparing a full application. When putting together an LOI, it is important to emphasize the clinical significance of your research, the study population you will be examining, the sample size, the plans for the intervention and analysis, as well as your anticipated results. Make your LOI as compelling as possible. If your topic is not considered compelling by the agency, they will not ask you for a full application. Closely examine their LOI request, since they often have specific criteria for the proposal. Tailor your LOI so that it closely meets their stated criteria.

Career Awards

Career awards (also known as career development or salary support awards) provide funds to help pay your salary. Obtaining one of these grants helps protect your time for research activities. These awards are often available only to new or mid-career investigators. Career awards are available from federal funding agencies such as the NIH, the CIHR, or from program-specific agencies such as the American Heart Association or the Heart and Stroke Foundation of Canada. Salary support can also be obtained from some state and provincial funding agencies.

United States

The United States and Canada have slightly different systems for funding the salaries of physician-scientists. In the United States, when you are awarded an operating grant, you are allowed to devote a portion of the budget to your salary and the salaries of your co-investigators. There are specific criteria regulating what portion of the budget can be devoted to salaries, and there is a salary cap determined by Congress each year. If you are a principal investigator or a co-investigator on one or more operating grants, you can "buy your way out" of clinical time by devoting a percentage of the budgets of these grants to your salary. The 2010 salary cap was $199,700.

In the United States, you can also obtain career awards such as Training Grants (T Series), Fellowship Funding Opportunities (F Series), and Career Development Awards (K Series) (Appendix 3). The K Series includes the KO1 Mentored Research Scientist Development Award, the KO2 Independent Scientist Award, and others. These awards provide direct salary support to physician-scientists. They are generally focused on supporting new investigators or mid-career or senior investigators who want to change their research focus.

Canada

In Canada, the career award is the primary mechanism for supporting the salaries of physician-scientists. Investigators in Canada cannot use any funds from operating grants for salary support for themselves or co-investigators. They can use the budget to pay the salaries of personnel such as research assistants and laboratory technicians. For this reason, physician-scientists apply for career awards. Career awards are usually awarded for blocks of three–five years. As you become more senior, the competition for career awards becomes more intense. Typically, a career award will only pay a portion of your salary. In my case, my career award pays approximately 25% of my salary. Because I spend 50% of my time doing research, my cardiology division covers the difference. Some Canadian investigators are supplemented by their division, their department, or the research institute of their hospital.

The amount of salary support varies from organization to organization. It depends on the seniority of the applicant and how much time they devote to research activities. One year before the termination of your career award, you will need to apply for the next grant up the ladder. The more senior you are, the more difficult it is to obtain salary support.

Grants for salary support are usually available for a total of 10–15 years. By the end of that time, if you are still a productive researcher, you will hopefully have received tenure (if available at your university). Tenure means that once salary support grants are no longer available, the university is responsible for paying a portion of your salary for the remainder of your career at the university. If you do not receive tenure or if it is not available at your institution, other arrangements can be made so that you can continue to conduct research. Your salary may be supplemented by your institution or you may be awarded a chair, for example.

It is important to note that for most Canadian physician-scientists, the majority of their salary does not come from salary support awards. Rather, it usually comes from clinical earnings and from additional supplementation received from the division, department, or research institute.

Applying for a Career Award

In the following two chapters, I discuss some of the specifics about how to structure an application for an operating grant. In this section, I discuss how to structure a proposal for a career award. Your application for a career award needs to be different from your application for operating funds. An application for operating funds is evaluated largely on the merits of the project itself, as well as the likelihood that the group of investigators you put together will be able to conduct the project. An application for a career award takes into account other factors. You need to be cognizant of these factors when putting together your application for a career award. I have served on several committees that review grant applications for career awards. When reviewing applications from junior physician-scientists, one funding agency provided guidelines suggesting that we take the following factors into consideration and assign them the following weights:

Training 20%
Grants, publications, and productivity 30%
Research milieu 10%
Autonomy and independence of research program 5%
Program of research 35%

Note that the research program only made up 35% of the overall score. As a result, when preparing your own career award applications, make sure that your proposal clearly documents the other factors that the review committee takes into consideration.

Training

It helps to have excellent and extensive training at well-known institutions. The more research training you receive, the more likely you will be to succeed as a physician-scientist. Review committees know this and take it into consideration when evaluating career award applications. Similarly, having additional degrees that demonstrate your commitment to research and the depth of your research knowledge is clearly a plus.

Productivity

Productivity is very important. Even if your proposed research program is flawless, unless you have demonstrated an ability to publish and obtain grants as a principal investigator, you might not receive a career award. Some slack is given to very junior candidates in terms of grant support, but they must have an excellent publication record and show that they have recently submitted grant applications and are waiting for results. In terms of publications, strive to have a minimum of one first author publication per year. Many abstracts and few publications is a bad sign. Having multiple publications related to your Masters or PhD thesis and no subsequent independent publications is also not auspicious. Having a few publications in high-impact journals is much more valuable than having many publications in low-impact journals. If you have many grants and few publications, this will also be viewed unfavorably. It is favorable for junior applicants to demonstrate that they have received small internal grants from their institutions. However, senior applicants need to demonstrate an ability to attract serious consistent funding from peer-reviewed agencies.

Research Milieu

It is important to indicate that you are located in a center where there is substantial support for research. Clearly state the amount of protected time you have for research. You should also discuss the roles and expertise of your co-investigators and the availability of equipment, research assistants, students, secretary, office space, computers, etc. The grant review committee needs to be convinced that your research program is feasible in the environment at your institution.

Autonomy/Independence

Members of the review committee also need to be convinced that you have what it takes to be a principal investigator. They need to see that you have been a first and senior author on publications and that you have been the principal applicant on funded grants from peer-reviewed organizations. Demonstrate to them that you have a history of being the initiator and originator of original research projects and that you are capable of conducting research projects from A to Z. Always being a co-investigator or a site investigator does not merit salary support.

Research Program

The research program is still the most important component of your application for a career award. The research question must be compelling and be of major clinical, public health, or scientific interest. If the question is not viewed as compelling, the best-written application will not be funded. As opposed to applications for operating funds (which focus on a single project), applications for career awards discuss a series of related projects (three is optimal). These projects should be given approximately equal weight and space in the application. Less than 50% of the description of a project and perhaps only 25–30% should be devoted to background. Adequate details about the research design need to be provided for each of the projects included in the application. The application should be well organized and readable. Avoid abbreviations that are not common. Make sure reasonable weight is given to the rationale, pilot study, study design, sample size and power issues, and plans for analysis. Studies should be ambitious but feasible. If they are outside your field of expertise, make sure the committee knows that you will be including co-investigators with experience in these areas. Do not waste space with lots of tables and figures. Avoid long, complex paragraphs. Use all the space available. Fill empty space with details of the proposed studies. Most reviewers will not have experience in your area of research. As a result, the research proposal must be organized and explained in simple terms. Sample size and power calculations should be easily replicated by the reviewers. Limit the number of hypotheses – three is ideal, seven is excessive. Hypotheses, objectives, and primary and secondary endpoints should all be presented in parallel. Define your primary and secondary endpoints. Finally, the duration of your proposed research program should match the duration of the career award you are applying for.

Summary

The ability to obtain peer-reviewed grant support is critical to your success as a new physician-scientist. There are many potential sources of funding; be aware of these sources and their guidelines. You can improve your chances of obtaining a grant by being aware of the RFAs and PAs announced by the funding agencies. It is important to note that the structure of an application for a career award is different from that of an application for operating funds. A career award application details a research program that involves several interrelated studies. Besides providing details of your proposed research program, be sure to document other pertinent elements like training, productivity, research milieu, and autonomy.

Key Points

- Choose the appropriate funding agency for your grant application.
- The NIH and CIHR are the primary federal funding agencies in the US and Canada, respectively.
- State, provincial, and local agencies are also possible sources of funding.
- Foundations typically fund proposals related their specific areas of interest.
- Industry support can be helpful but should not make up the bulk of your funding.
- Formulate a compelling research question with high clinical, public health, or scientific impact.
- Responding to RFAs and PAs can enhance your chances of obtaining funding.
- A career award will help protect your research time.

- While the decision to fund operating grants is largely based on your research question and study design, the decision to fund career awards is also dependent on your productivity, research milieu, training, and autonomy.

Suggested Reading

1. Burroughs Wellcome Fund and Howard Hughes Medical Institute. Making the Right Moves: A Practical Guide to Scientific Management for Postdocs and New Faculty. 2nd ed. Research Triangle Park, NC; Chevy Chase, MD: Burroughs Wellcome Fund; Howard Hughes Medical Institute; 2006.
2. Brand RA, Hannafin JA. The environment of the successful clinician-scientist. Clin Orthop Relat Res 2006; 449: 67–71.
3. Canadian Institutes of Health Research. www.cihr.ca. Accessed March 30, 2010.
4. Inouye SK, Fiellin DA. An evidence-based guide to writing grant proposals for clinical research. Ann Intern Med 2005; 142: 274–282.
5. Johnson VE. Statistical analysis of the National Institutes of Health peer review system. Proc Natl Acad Sci USA 2008; 105: 11076–11080.
6. Johnston SC, Hauser SL. Peer review at National Institutes of Health: small steps forward. Ann Neurol 2008; 64: A15–A17.
7. Kaiser J. National Institutes of Health. Two strikes and you're out, grant applicants learn. Science 2008; 322: 358.
8. Mandel HG, Vesell ES. Declines in funding of NIH R01 research grants. Science 2006; 313: 1387–1388.
9. National Institutes of Health. www.nih.gov. Accessed March 30, 2010.
10. National Institutes of Health. Types of Grant Programs. http://grants.nih.gov/grants/oer.htm. Accessed May 7, 2009.
11. Rothman DJ, McDonald WJ, Berkowitz CD, et al. Professional medical associations and their relationships with industry: a proposal for controlling conflict of interest. JAMA 2009; 301: 1367–1372.
12. Urrutia R. Academic skills: a concise guide to grant writing. Pancreatology 2007; 7: 307–310.
13. Vastag B. Increasing R01 competition concerns researchers. J Natl Cancer Inst 2006; 98: 1436–1438.

Chapter 12
Grantsmanship

*Donors don't give to institutions. They invest in ideas and
people in whom they believe.*

–G. T. Smith

Introduction

This chapter is long on strategy and short on science. It may sound calculating to
you, but that is not my intention. I assume that you love science, research, and the
creation of new knowledge. However, you need funding to pursue these interests.
A solid knowledge of the strategies that can improve your chances of obtaining
funding is essential. In this chapter, I discuss the following topics: (1) identifying a
fundable topic; (2) choosing the right funding agency and committee; (3) establishing a strong research team; (4) putting together a realistic budget; and (5) employing
strategies that will improve your chances of obtaining funding. Good grantsmanship
is a critical skill that you need to develop early in your career.

Identifying a Fundable Topic

One of the most important determinants of your success as a physician-scientist is
your ability to identify fundable topics to research. This issue requires considerable
thought. You will spend many hours putting together a grant proposal on the topic
you choose. If you obtain funding, you will spend a year or more on the project. As
a result, you need to identify a feasible, compelling topic of scientific interest that
will be of major interest to a funding agency and that will retain your interest as
well.

Compelling Topics

Compelling topics are those that are cutting edge and that have public health impact
and significant relevance to patients. A compelling research question is applicable

M.J. Eisenberg, *The Physician Scientist's Career Guide*,
DOI 10.1007/978-1-60327-908-6_12, © Springer Science+Business Media, LLC 2011

to patient care and clinical outcomes. It has novel mechanistic insights, a fresh approach to an old problem, or major public health consequences.

New physician-scientists often have fixed ideas about what they want to study. These ideas are natural extensions of their clinical exposure as medical students, residents, and fellows and of their additional research training. However, early in your career you may find that what you want to study is not what the funding agencies are funding. If your topic is not of particular interest to the funding agencies, it will be difficult to obtain financial support for your research. Although you may acquire modest sums of money for your research, it will require many revisions and resubmissions of your grant applications. If this is the case, it may be more strategic to modify your topic so that it is more in line with the priorities of the funding agencies.

Rather than jumping into a grant proposal with the first idea you have, consider multiple potential topics and whether they are compelling research questions or not. Keep an eye out for hot topics when attending conferences, reading the recent literature, and in discussions with colleagues; this will give you a good idea of what agencies are interested in funding. It is also useful to check the websites of funding agencies to see what topics and types of projects they have funded over the past few years.

Once you have an idea for a project, perform a quick literature search on Medline. This will allow you to assess the status of your topic. You will quickly determine if too much has been done on this particular topic or if it is innovative and novel. Once you develop a list of topics that seem both feasible and innovative, run them by your colleagues to see whether other investigators think these ideas are interesting. You need to enter a grant competition with a well-written grant on a clinically relevant and highly compelling topic. Do not take a moderately interesting topic and try to make it into something that it is not.

Scope of Proposal

Keep in mind that you need to generate publishable research findings within three–five years of your appointment as assistant professor. For this reason, do not be too ambitious. A large randomized clinical trial that will take five years to complete and longer to publish is probably not appropriate for an initial grant submission. It is not uncommon for new physician-scientists to be overly ambitious when submitting their first few grant applications. I caution you against this. At the same time, do not choose a topic that is too limited in scope. The best way to assess the scope of your proposal is to run it by your more experienced colleagues. Do this as early as possible so that you do not put a lot of time and effort into a proposal that your colleagues do not think will be successful. Get a senior investigator to review your proposal early enough in the process that he or she has enough time to help you reshape it.

Making Your Case

To decide whether your topic is compelling enough to be funded, you need to think like the members of a grant review committee. They are presented with many grants to review and will fund at most the top 25%. Your idea needs to stand out from the rest. Make it obvious on the first page of the proposal how compelling your topic is. The significance of the research question needs to be emphasized at the very beginning of the application, at the end of the background section, and again at the conclusion of the proposal. I cannot stress how important it is to make this clear to the reviewers.

Structure

The research question needs to be broken down concisely and accurately into hypotheses, objectives, and endpoints, so that a reader can quickly figure out what you want to study, how you will study it, and why it is important. You will most likely have several hypotheses, each of which should have a corresponding objective and endpoint. For example, if one hypothesis were that a given drug increases abstinence from smoking at one year in a given population, then the corresponding objective would be to measure the effect of this drug in this population at one year. The corresponding endpoint would be smoking abstinence at one year, as measured by whatever tool you select as being the most effective. Secondary and tertiary endpoints might involve assessing safety, effectiveness, cost effectiveness, quality of life, or additional biological measures. Usually, there are at least three hypotheses with parallel objectives and endpoints. Limit yourself to five hypotheses at the most; a common mistake made by new investigators is to be too ambitious and to try to investigate everything in one grant. This is another reason why it is very helpful to show your grant applications to more experienced investigators early in the process; as a result, you will get an idea of whether your proposed study is reasonable in scope.

Hypotheses, objectives, and endpoints should be presented in parallel order so that is easy for a reviewer to understand which steps apply to which question. This is the crux of your proposal; what you want to discover and how you will study it. Therefore, it is essential to make this very clear to your readers. State these ideas in your one-page summary and in the background section of your proposal. The rest of the proposal should relate back to these statements, explaining in detail what has been done already, what you are going to do, how it will improve knowledge and patient care, and so on. Committee members need to be enthralled and impressed with your proposal right from the beginning.

Ultimately, if your research question is not compelling, your grant will not be funded, no matter how good your research design or how strong your investigative team. I am not saying that you should not pursue your research ideas; just that if you find it difficult to get your ideas funded, you may need to reframe your research question or even redirect your research program to a more fundable topic. However, I do not wish to overstate the case. Although it is important to consider what the funding agencies are interested in, that does not mean you can only research those areas. You might still obtain funding even if your topic is not a priority area for the agency, providing your idea is innovative and impactful and your proposal is well-written. Be strategic and consider how to make your topic compelling to the committee.

Feasibility

In addition to being compelling, your proposal needs to be feasible. Even if you have the most compelling idea in the world, if the committee does not think it is feasible, they will not fund it. Feasibility implies that the topic lends itself to study and that you have the tools, skills, and time required to study the question. If you decide to study a particular aspect of a very rare disease, demonstrate that you have access to patients with that disease. If you have only a handful of these patients at your institution, you need to demonstrate that investigators at other institutions who do have access to these patients will be collaborating with you.

As you become more experienced, your projects and proposals can become more ambitious. However, never lose sight of the importance of the feasibility of your projects. If, for example, you are putting together a large, multi-center, randomized controlled trial, you need to demonstrate the following:

- That you have access to the requisite patients or to sites where investigators are willing to enroll patients for you.
- That you have access to the drug (and the placebo if indicated) or the intervention in question.
- That other investigators are willing to enroll patients for the amount of money that you propose for reimbursement.
- That you have a well-rounded group of investigators who can supervise the project.
- That you have the data management capabilities to run a project of this scope.

To document these important factors, include letters of collaboration from investigators who are willing to enroll patients for you. It is helpful if they can provide information about the number of patients with the relevant condition who have been treated at their institution in the past year or two. This gives the grant committee an idea of whether you are likely to meet the necessary enrollment numbers for your study with your collaborating sites. You and your co-investigators should demonstrate your ability to perform the study in the feasibility section of your grant proposal and in your CV modules. Ideally, include pilot study data to show that you have already successfully enrolled patients and met objectives in a small sample of patients. This shows that your proposal is feasible and that your team has the capacity to conduct the study.

In addition, it is important to demonstrate that you have the required experience to conduct the study. Your grant proposal may be the most ambitious that you have presented yet, but your track record should show that you have successfully conducted smaller studies of a similar nature that have given you the experience to conduct this study. If you are proposing a study in an area for which you do not have substantial experience, you need to demonstrate that your co-investigators have the required experience. If you submit a well-written, well-conceived genetics application, but no one on your research team has any experience with genetics studies, the committee will conclude that your proposal is not feasible for your team.

The answers to the above issues may seem obvious to you, but they may not be obvious to committee members. Therefore, they must be clearly addressed in your application. You may have the most compelling idea ever presented to a review committee, but unless you can demonstrate feasibility, they will not fund your study. To make it clear that your study is feasible, document and highlight that you have the necessary resources and qualified personnel to carry it out successfully.

Public Health or Clinical Impact

In addition to identifying a compelling topic that is of interest to you and to the review committee, it is important to identify a topic that is of significant public health or clinical importance. Obscure topics, or those that are not likely to generate knowledge that will improve patient care in the near future, are a lower priority for funding agencies than topics that might have significant public health impact in the near future. As a result, if you have some latitude in choosing your topic, try to choose one that is a major health issue.

For example, there is a growing obesity epidemic across the globe and in North America in particular. The profound implications this epidemic will have on patterns of disease over the next few decades are well recognized. This is clearly an area of high priority for funding agencies. Any topic that relates to the obesity epidemic is more likely to be funded than an obscure topic with little immediate clinical relevance. Even if your topic is more basic science than clinical, if you can relate it to the growing obesity epidemic, you are more likely to get it funded. It is essential that you make your proposal's relevance to patient care and public health very clear in the introduction and conclusion sections of your proposal. The committee will be examining many proposals and they need to consider yours a high priority for you to obtain funding.

Competition

When choosing topics for grant applications, consider whether other research teams are engaged in the same research. It is not ideal to choose a compelling research idea that is identical to one being pursued by larger, more experienced research teams than yours. These groups can put together a study, complete it, and publish it well before you can get your grant proposal funded. Identify a topic that is feasible and compelling but that will not face major competition in the immediate future. This will allow you to complete the project and publish it without being "scooped." This is an important consideration for new physician-scientists. This does not mean that you need to avoid hot topics for which there is already a lot of research in progress; it just means that you need to hone your idea so that it is a very specific question that is not being widely studied. Approach a topic from a different angle than other teams have taken.

Often, new investigators want to pursue an area they were working on with their supervisors during their advanced research training. However, their supervisors may still be investigating that topic. Be clear with the review committee that you are independent from your supervisor. If you are going to study the same topic, get a letter from your supervisor stating that they are no longer going to study this topic and that this topic is now yours alone. If your supervisor is going to continue to study this topic, and if you wish to pursue it as well, you should pick a different angle to study. It is quite likely that your supervisor will be able to collect the data, analyze it, and publish a paper well before you get underway. When thinking about a topic for grant submission, choose one that is compelling and sufficiently ambitious but that will allow you to publish some meaningful data without much competition over the next few years.

Funding Agencies, Guidelines, and Committees

You need to be very familiar with the funding agencies, their guidelines for grant submissions, and their committees. Visit agency websites on a regular basis and read the applicable instructions and guidelines. Familiarize yourself with the guidelines at least two months before the actual submission. The first time you submit a grant application to a given agency, you will find it to be a tedious and time-consuming process (see Table 12.1 for tips on how to get started). However, you need to read and reread the guidelines. If you do not follow the instructions, your grant will be rejected without review. There are numerous application guidelines that must be followed. These range from registration deadlines, to the points your proposal must touch on, to the number of appendices allowed. Your proposal needs to address all the elements that a particular competition requires (Table 12.2); different information and a different structure are required for various types of competitions and agencies. There are also formatting requirements for margins, font size, headers and footers, and the maximum number of pages allowed. If you wait until the last minute to read these guidelines and instructions, it is unlikely that you will be able to thoroughly adhere to them in your application. There are also many forms to fill out. You can have a secretary or a research assistant help with filling out the forms, but you need to go over each one of them in detail before the grant is submitted.

Table 12.1 Getting started on your grant proposal

Do a preliminary literature search to establish feasibility and relevance of possible topics
Choose a topic
Choose a funding agency and committee
Check the website of the institution for general guidelines and those specific to your competition
Consider the skills your co-investigators need to have for the project to be successful
Approach potential co-investigators and collaborators via e-mail, phone, letter
Discuss the details of the collaboration – frequency of meetings, publications, etc.
Get everyone involved in developing the study design and grant application
If needed, register your proposal before submitting
Find out what signatures you will need from co-investigators, institution heads, etc.
Create a lay summary
Prepare a one-page summary early on
Research previous studies and background information for inclusion in the proposal
Find out if you will need to mail an application or submit it online
Circulate a well-edited draft of the proposal among the co-investigators for comments
Address any comments that are useful/feasible and re-circulate

Table 12.2 Typical components of an operating grant proposal[1]

Supplementary documents

• Funding agency forms
• One-page summary
• Lay summary
• Summary of progress
• Response to reviewers

The proposal

1.	Title	
2.	Hypothesis	
3.	Objectives	Overall and specific
4.	Background	Introduction to subject
		Previous studies
		Pilot data
		Significance
5.	Rationale	
6.	Study design	Type of study
		Population, intervention/exposure, duration of follow-up
		Sample size/power calculations
		Data analysis
		Potential benefits/risks
7.	Organization/project management	Institution
		Role/qualifications of principal investigator
		Role/qualifications of co-investigators, collaborators, staff
8.	Limitations	
9.	Feasibility	
10.	Significance	
11.	References	

Table 12.2 (continued)

12. Appendices	Research ethics board (REB) approval and letter
	Case report forms (CRFs) and consent forms
	Pilot data
	Tables and figures
	Letters of collaboration
	Detailed timeline
13. Budget and budget justification	
14. CV modules and attachments of principal and co-investigators	

[1] The items required and the order of items may differ for different types of studies and for different funding agencies.

Choosing the Right Funding Agency

Choosing the right funding agency is critical to your chances of being funded. Submitting a grant proposal related to colon cancer to the American Heart Association is not likely to be successful. Most senior physician-scientists are funded by only one or two funding agencies. As a new physician-scientist, you need to identify the funding agencies that are most likely to fund your type of research. The most common funding agencies in the United States and Canada are the National Institutes of Health (NIH) and the Canadian Institutes of Health Research (CIHR), respectively (for lists of NIH and CIHR grants, see Appendices 3 and 4). However, your particular area may be of interest to a topic-specific funding agency. If you are studying a cardiovascular topic, the American Heart Association might be a good funding agency to explore. If you are investigating topics related to cancer, the American Cancer Society might be an appropriate agency to consider. It is common practice to send a grant proposal simultaneously to different funding agencies. However, if you are fortunate enough to be funded by more than one agency, you will have to choose which award to accept.

When you are putting together your proposal, be aware of the requirements of each of the funding agencies to which you are submitting. Some agencies have quite different instructions concerning what should be included in a proposal and how it should be organized. It is not a pleasant experience to discover, right before the submission deadline, that you have to substantially revise the content or format of your proposal. Keep your work to a minimum and familiarize yourself with the requirements early in the process.

When selecting the most appropriate funding agencies, you need to check their websites. Often, recipients of grants from previous competitions are listed. You can look at the funded investigators and their topics. If none of the topics are similar to yours, this might not be the right funding agency for you. You also need to examine the amount of money that each funding agency typically awards. This is sometimes listed on their website along with previous award recipients and their topics. The website will announce the maximum amount that the funding agency awards. For example, they may award a maximum of $200,000 per year for no more than five years. You need to know this from the beginning so that you can develop your proposal accordingly. You can submit a proposal that has a larger budget than a given funding agency will provide for. However, if you do so, make it clear in your proposal that you are submitting to multiple funding agencies in order to procure complementary funding. In summary, when deciding which funding agency to submit to, examine whether the agency has funded topics like yours in the past, whether the amount of money they award is appropriate to the magnitude of your project, and whether the agency is likely to find your topic compelling.

Choosing the Right Committee

Funding agencies usually have multiple committees that review grants. You need to submit your grant to the appropriate committee. If your grant is a clinical cardiovascular study and you submit it to a committee that reviews only basic science studies, it is unlikely to receive funding. If you are lucky, the funding agency will note the discrepancy and redirect your grant to the correct committee. However, you cannot count on this, and it is your responsibility to select the appropriate committee. Often, a particular grant application could potentially be submitted to several committees. For example, an application that proposes to use a large administrative database to examine whether a particular drug causes a rare cardiovascular outcome could be submitted to a clinical cardiovascular committee or a population science committee. Think carefully about which committee will give you the best chance of being funded. If your application is submitted to a clinical cardiovascular committee, it will be in competition with many clinical studies, and the committee may not have the methodological expertise to review your proposal. It might fit in better with the goals and aims of the population science committee.

Each funding agency has a program officer associated with each committee who deals with principal investigators submitting grant proposals. After you put together a one-page grant summary, it is well worthwhile for you to speak with a program officer at your targeted funding agency. Tell this individual that you are a new investigator preparing a grant proposal. Tell them the topic of your grant proposal and ask them what committee they think it would be best to submit to. It is always useful to study the websites of the funding agencies to see what types of grants the different committees have funded. If your study uses a particular methodology, it may need to go to a particular committee. For example, any study involving randomization of patients may need to be submitted to a randomized controlled trials committee, regardless of the subject matter. If an agency functions this way, it would be a mistake to submit an application involving randomization of patients to another committee. Your application may be redirected to the randomized controlled trials committee, but might also be rejected and returned to you. You will then have to wait until the next submission period to resubmit to the correct committee. Therefore, carefully consider which committee you send your proposal to.

You may have put together an excellent and compelling grant proposal, but you will have a smaller chance of being funded by some committees than others, even if your proposal is technically relevant to each of them. In addition to studying the descriptions of each committee, it is always helpful to speak to more senior investigators who have experience in this area. Furthermore, speak to the program officers of the committees you are considering. These individuals will be more than happy to discuss the nature of your proposal and which committee to send it to.

Establishing a Strong Research Team

As a new investigator, you are an untested product. It is important that you put together the right team for each grant proposal so that the grant review committee is convinced that you have the expertise to complete the project in a timely fashion. Obtain support from the right co-investigators and collaborators for your project. I discussed this issue in detail in Chapter 8 in the context of getting your research program off the ground. Below, I discuss this issue in the context of your first few grant applications.

Choosing the Right Co-Investigators

You will benefit from the inclusion of experienced co-investigators who can review and comment on your grant application before you submit it. These individuals often have helpful suggestions that will substantially improve your proposal. Provide them with a draft of your proposal and sufficient time for them to review it and for you to incorporate their suggestions before submission to the funding agency. Make sure that these individuals are truly engaged in the process from the beginning. They should be involved in the conception of the question, writing sections of the grant proposal, and reviewing the proposal prior to submission.

A strong research team is an important element that demonstrates to the review committee that your study is feasible. When the committee sees a diverse team with complementary strengths, they will have greater confidence that your team will be able to complete the research project. It is not helpful to have multiple team members with the same qualifications. Instead, each individual should offer different strengths and expertise. When I conduct randomized controlled trials, for example, I provide the clinical background and epidemiology expertise. To supplement my areas of expertise, I include a biostatistician, a PhD epidemiologist, a pure clinician with substantive subject knowledge in the area, and others if their skills are required. I have been awarded several grants for research in the area of smoking cessation. To complement my skills in these grant applications, I included a respirologist, a PhD epidemiologist with experience in the area, a biostatistician, a public health expert, and a knowledge translation expert. Each of these individuals brings a different set of skills and strengths to the table.

When you submit your grant application, you will be required to include a CV module for each co-investigator. These CVs are examined less closely than yours by the committee. Nevertheless, committee members want to see that your co-investigators will bring added value to the research team. To increase your chances of success, these sections need to be as impressive as possible. Consider the needs of the project and choose the necessary team members well in advance, so that each of them has time to prepare a comprehensive and professional CV module. It is not enough for your team to possess the skills to complete the project; they need to demonstrate this to the committee very clearly.

Choosing the Right Collaborators

In contrast to co-investigators, collaborators are not required to provide a CV when you submit your grant application. Instead, collaborators provide letters of collaboration, which are appended to the application. These letters need to demonstrate enthusiasm and moderately detailed knowledge of the subject matter of the application. I have reviewed grant applications in which letters of collaboration from different individuals were included, but in which the wording of the letters was exactly the same. It was clear that the principal investigator requested a letter of collaboration and provided a template to all collaborators. This practice is not viewed favorably by review committees. Instead, letters of collaboration should be unique, should be from individuals who have the potential to add value to the application, and who demonstrate knowledge of and enthusiasm for the proposal.

Other Team-Related Issues

You need to examine the team from the point of view of the review committee. Are the individuals strong researchers in their own right? Do they each have a history of high-quality publications? Are they authorities in their field? Do they have the necessary skills that will help advance the project? How will the team collaborate if they are not in the same geographical area? Although it might be helpful to have one or two team members who do not have much of a track record in research but who have a lot of practical knowledge about the subject, the majority of the members should be established researchers. The team needs to be productive and work toward a common goal. The responsibilities of each member should be described in the grant proposal. This should not be an extensive section but it should provide a breakdown of their responsibilities in a few short sentences.

Budgets

For most funding agencies, the budget of your project will not be a major factor in deciding whether or not to fund your grant proposal. Usually, grant review committees examine the scientific aspects of your proposal and recommend a score independent of the budget. Once the scoring is done, however, the committee will then examine the budget.

Most members of grant review committees are experienced investigators. Having put together many grant proposals themselves, they are very familiar with budgets. They will quickly notice if you have "padded" your budget. If your budget is padded, the committee might recommend that the amount awarded be substantially reduced. They will also recognize if you have not fully appreciated the costs involved in a study of the scope presented. In this case, the committee will not increase the budget, but will instead send the grant back to you for revision to make it more feasible. You can respond by increasing the budget or decreasing the scope of your project. It is worth noting that if this occurs, your proposal is not considered accepted pending revision of the budget – you will have to revise the budget and resubmit the entire proposal at the next competition. Though a committee may be willing to fund your study, a budget that is not sufficiently comprehensive or well justified may prevent you from receiving the funding. In addition, there is a chance that if you resubmit, your proposal will not be accepted the next time around, so it is crucial to get your budget right the first time.

Make-Up of a Budget

The budget information for a grant application usually has two components: the budget itself and the budget justification. The budget is a line item list of all the components and costs organized by year. For example, the budget of a randomized controlled trial might include data management, drugs, materials, personnel, travel and other costs. For each component, you list the individual items in that area and their costs. Under personnel, for example, you should list your coordinator, your secretary, the research nurses at each of the collaborating institutions, and the computer programmer, with their respective salaries and benefits. You also need to indicate whether they are full- or part-time.

Each year should have its own section. If you are requesting funding for five years, the salary and benefits for each of the above personnel may be repeated five times, once each year. List a subtotal for each year and a total for the entire project. The more detailed the budget, the more likely you are to receive the requested funds. The reviewers need to see that you are realistic about the costs involved in conducting your research. Carefully consider the personnel, equipment, administrative, travel, and service costs that are likely to occur, as well as other costs that might arise. If you have not put together a budget before, obtain copies of several grant proposals that have been funded in the past. Examine their budgets closely and emulate them.

The budget justification is a separate section describing the budget items in narrative form. This section is often several pages long. At the beginning of the budget justification, there is usually an introductory paragraph detailing the yearly costs as well as the overall costs for the project. You should also provide the total costs for each of the major components, such as personnel, materials, drugs, etc. Following this introductory paragraph, include detailed paragraphs about each major component of the budget. For example, if a large part of the budget is costs attributable to research nurses, explain how many hours will be required for each of them and how their time will be spent. How many hours will the research nurse spend enrolling patients? Filling out baseline case report forms? Making follow-up telephone calls? Conducting follow-up visits? etc. Include as much detail as possible in the budget justification. The committee needs to see that you are realistic about the number of hours and the amount of equipment and materials required for your research.

Duration

Study duration is important. Try to have your proposal funded for as long as possible so that you have the time and the funding to complete your objectives. Typically, funding agencies do not fund for less than one year or for more than five years. Be realistic about how much time your project will require. Do not ask for five years of funding for a project that can be done in one year. On the other hand, do not truncate your study timeline with the idea that it will be more attractive to a funding agency. It is better to ask for what you need than to scale it down to make your proposal more attractive. Request the duration and amount of funding that will make it possible for you to succeed, no more and no less. Physician-scientists tend to be overly ambitious with their proposals and budgets. It is more important to get a less expensive proposal funded on the first or second try than it is to get an ambitious, very expensive grant proposal funded after years of resubmissions.

During your first few years as a physician-scientist, submit modest but compelling grant proposals with modest but realistic budgets. When review committees see that you are a new investigator with an interesting, feasible idea that is not too costly, they will be more inclined to fund your project. If you present a costly and ambitious proposal, it is less likely that they will fund you. Because you are an unknown quantity as a researcher, they will be concerned about your ability to complete such a project and will not want to invest huge sums of money over a long period of time until you have a more extensive track record.

Committee Considerations

Peer review committees typically discuss the budget, including the duration of funding. If an investigator submits a grant that is considered excellent scientifically but the research team's productivity has been low, the committee may decide to reduce the duration of the funding or the amount funded. They usually discuss what parts of the budget could be reduced to save money. The personnel requested by the investigators are considered with particular interest. Many grants are top-heavy with personnel requests. Documentation of the materials and supplies will also be examined. I have seen some of these expenses cut as well. This is particularly common if one of the committee members has experience in the area and is familiar with the specific resources required. At one particular grant review committee meeting,

I attended, grants were typically funded at $100,000–$150,000 per year for three–five years. If the funding request exceeded $200,000 per year, that budget was examined very closely. There were very few applications that requested less than $100,000 per year.

Funding Agency Guidelines

In addition to accounting for the costs of your study, it is also important that your budget takes into account the amount the committee and funding agency are likely to award. There are typically rules about the duration of funding, the total amount, the maximum amount per year, and what the funds can be used for. For example, NIH-funded investigators can use a portion of their grants to augment their salary; this is not true in all countries. Similarly, some agencies restrict the amount of funding you can use for secretarial support or equipment. It is critical that you familiarize yourself with these rules or your proposal might be rejected without review. To do this, carefully read the regulations on the agency and committee websites. You should also review the previous awards from this committee and agency. If they have never awarded over $200,000 per year, make sure that you ask for less than this.

In terms of your research career and promotion, you need to demonstrate research productivity and grant support within three–five years of receiving your first academic appointment. For this reason, you need to obtain your first operating grant as soon as possible. Even a small grant will allow you to put together a research team and get your program off the ground, after which you can work on obtaining more substantial support. To ensure that you have continuous funding from the start, put considerable thought into the budget of every grant proposal that you submit.

Strategies for Success

The current funding climate in North America is not good. This means that even if your grant is excellent, it may not be funded. However, there are several strategies you can employ that will increase your chances of being funded.

Targeting Smaller Agencies

One strategy that can be useful in helping you get your first few grants funded is that of targeting smaller agencies. Although your application may be less compelling to major agencies like the NIH, it may be very appealing to smaller agencies that have more focused interests. These agencies often offer smaller awards than federal agencies. However, a small grant from a small agency can help you develop pilot data that can substantially improve the impact of subsequent submissions to larger funding agencies. As a result, explore smaller agencies within your area of interest.

Each university and research institute keeps an extensive list of relevant funding agencies. They periodically circulate these lists to their physician-scientists. If you are not already on this e-mail list, you need to be. There is often a department of grants within your university that keeps track of this information. Contact them and ask to be informed of the different funding opportunities available. Both the university and your research institute will typically circulate by e-mail any requests for proposals sent by the different agencies; read them in detail. The more information you have, the more likely it is that you will identify a likely source of funding.

Sub-Studies of Trials in Progress

A strategy that is often successful is to submit a proposal for a sub-study. If a large multi-center trial has already been funded, propose a sub-study that can be done in conjunction with the larger trial. For example, in a study that randomizes patients to one drug versus another and follows long-term clinical outcomes, submit a sub-study proposal to analyze blood that was already banked for genetic analyses. You could then associate the genotypes with the clinical outcomes and interactions with the drug. A prospective study of this nature might be prohibitively expensive. However, because the main study has already been funded, the patients have been enrolled, and the blood is already collected, it will require a lot less funding to perform your proposed study. The funding agency will get added value by funding your sub-study, and you will be able to explore an extremely compelling question at a relatively low cost.

Renewals

Submitting a renewal application is an important strategy for increasing your chances of being funded. You can apply for a renewal grant only if you have been previously funded by that agency. A renewal application is a request for a new grant for you to build on the knowledge gained during the first grant. The new study is a natural continuation of your previously funded work. You need to submit a renewal application before the termination of your current grant. Renewals are funded at a significantly higher rate than de novo proposals.

You should clearly indicate in the text and on the application forms that your grant is a renewal application. Make the connection between your earlier work and the proposed work very clear. Your new grant should be a natural continuation of the work that you have been doing. Do not use the same title as the previous grant, but the new title should be similar. One would typically expect to see many of the same co-investigators, since they were involved in your previous grant. The nature of the study should be somewhat similar. It is important that you demonstrate your productivity during the first grant and provide a detailed description of your progress to date. This description can include a summary of your findings and a list of articles and abstracts resulting from the previous project (published or in preparation), presentations attended, and training provided to students over the course of the project. You do not want to appear as though you are requesting more funding to complete objectives from the previous project. The renewal will be based on this work, but should have completely new objectives and questions.

When preparing your renewal application, keep in mind that your success at obtaining funding the first time does not guarantee that you will be successful with your renewal application. Some investigators assume that because their first grant was funded, the renewal application will be a formality and they will not need to spend a lot of time on it. This is definitely not the case. Spend just as much time preparing your renewal application as you did on your original proposal. Since you will need to formulate new objectives, hypotheses, and methodology, the same amount of work will be required as for the first time; you cannot just revise your previous application.

You usually have only one opportunity to obtain a renewal grant. Submit your renewal application six months to one year before the current grant expires. The idea is to have continuous funding from this agency so you can be maximally productive. If they reject your application and you resubmit it after your first grant has expired, you will probably need to submit it as a de novo application. However, some agencies allow you to submit one additional renewal application if the first one is unsuccessful. In this case, incorporate as many of the suggestions offered by the reviewers and include them in your response to them. Do this as quickly as possible so you can meet the next competition deadline. You will be unable to submit it as an "unsuccessful renewal application" if too much time has elapsed between the end of your previous grant and the resubmission.

A renewal application needs to demonstrate your commitment to the area, your productivity during the first grant, the feasibility of your new objectives, the continuing importance of the subject, and the strength of your research team. Use every strategy you have to be funded. A renewal application is an excellent way to help you beat the odds.

Summary

The ability to obtain funding for grant proposals is a critical skill for a new physician-scientist. Unfortunately, most physician-scientists have little training in this area. There are many strategies that you can employ to improve the likelihood of your grant being funded. Before you put together your proposal, discuss possible research questions with more senior colleagues. Obtain copies of previous successful grant applications and study them closely. Examine the websites of the funding agencies and the requirements of the particular committees to which you plan to submit. Collect as much information as possible before putting together your application, including pilot data if possible. Assemble a strong group of co-investigators and collaborators. Your ability to write winning grant applications will largely determine your success as a physician-scientist. You need to develop the necessary skills as quickly as possible.

Key Points

- Choose a topic that is compelling, feasible, and that has major public health or clinical impact.
- Choose a funding agency and committee that funds research similar to your proposed study.
- Do not be too ambitious; you need to publish findings within three–five years.
- Demonstrate the feasibility of your project in terms of personnel, resources, implementation, etc.
- Do not choose a topic on which other researchers will publish before you can.
- Run topics by senior colleagues before writing a proposal.
- Examine agency websites for guidelines and previous funding history.
- Put together a team whose skills are complementary.
- Be realistic about how much funding and time you need.
- Increase your chances of obtaining funding by targeting smaller funding agencies, submitting proposals for sub-studies, and submitting renewal applications.

Suggested Reading

1. Burroughs Wellcome Fund and Howard Hughes Medical Institute. Making the Right Moves: A Practical Guide to Scientific Management for Postdocs and New Faculty. 2nd ed. Research Triangle Park, NC; Chevy Chase, MD: Burroughs Wellcome Fund; Howard Hughes Medical Institute; 2006.
2. Adelstein SJ. Preparing a grant proposal. Invest Radiol 1993; 28 (Suppl 2): S10–S12.
3. Canadian Institutes of Health Research. Tips for writing a successful CIHR Grant Application or Request for Renewal. J Can Chiropr Assoc 2004; 48: 301–304.
4. Dyrbye LN, Lindor KD, LaRusso NF, Cook DA. Research productivity of graduates from 3 physician-scientist training programs. Am J Med 2008; 121: 1107–1113.
5. Greenspan RH. Grantsmanship. Invest Radiol 1993; 28 (Suppl 2): S3–S5.
6. Holcombe RF. Viewpoint: who's watching out for the clinical academician? Acad Med 2005; 80: 905–907.
7. Inouye SK, Fiellin DA. An evidence-based guide to writing grant proposals for clinical research. Ann Intern Med 2005; 142: 274–282.
8. Kundel HL, Walsh C. Preparing a research grant application budget. Invest Radiol 1993; 28 (Suppl 2): S13–S16.
9. Melnick A. Transitioning from fellowship to a physician-scientist career track. Hematol Am Soc Hematol Educ Program 2008; 2008: 16–22.
10. Thabane L, Thomas T, Ye C, Paul J. Posing the research question: not so simple. Can J Anaesth 2009; 56: 71–79.

Chapter 13
Peer Review of Grant Applications

You can have brilliant ideas, but if you can't get them across, your ideas won't get you anywhere.

–Lee Iacocca

Introduction

Although each funding agency has a slightly different method of conducting peer reviews of grant applications, the process at most agencies is largely similar. A good understanding of the review process will improve your grant proposals and consequently your chances of obtaining funding. In this chapter, I describe the peer review process at a particular funding agency for which I reviewed to give you an idea of the details of the process. The committee meeting I describe below occurred over one and a half days, during which we reviewed more than 50 grants. Following my description of the meeting, I provide some of the specific tips I have learned about preparing grant applications.

Committee Members

Sixteen committee members attended the meeting, including the Committee Chair and the Scientific Officer. The role of the Chair was to coordinate the discussion. The Scientific Officer was responsible for writing the Scientific Officer's notes, which were brief summaries of the committee's discussion of each submission. The Scientific Officer's notes contained the major comments of the reviewers and were subsequently delivered with the detailed reviews of the internal reviewers to the applicants. In addition to the members of the committee, two administrative members of the funding agency were present. Each committee member received a group of grants to review several months in advance of the meeting. I received 12 grants to review. I was the first reviewer on six, the second reviewer on three, and the reader on three.

M.J. Eisenberg, *The Physician Scientist's Career Guide*,
DOI 10.1007/978-1-60327-908-6_13, © Springer Science+Business Media, LLC 2011

Committee Discussions

During committee discussions, the first reviewer was responsible for providing a comprehensive account of the study rationale, the design, and the aspects of the proposal that were likely to affect funding. The first reviewer provided a detailed account of the principal investigator's CV, including qualifications, publication, and grant history. In addition, the first reviewer discussed the qualifications of the co-investigators and collaborators. He or she introduced the study by providing a detailed account of the rationale and study design. This included a review of the experiments to be performed, as well as sample size, power calculations, and plans for analysis. Finally, the reviewer presented major and minor criticisms of the application. This presentation took 10–15 minutes to complete. Following the presentation by the first reviewer, the second reviewer provided specific details or comments that were not covered by the first reviewer. This typically took about 5 minutes. When the second reviewer was finished presenting, the reader provided any additional comments not covered by the first two reviewers. After the presentations, there was a general discussion among committee members. Other members had electronic or hard copy versions of the grant application but in most cases did not have the opportunity to examine it in advance. In addition to the topics mentioned above, the committee also discussed the value that would be added by a particular study.

Half of the committee members were pure scientists and half were physician-scientists. The members possessed diverse knowledge and experience. Many of them did not have specific content knowledge about the particular grant topic under discussion. As a result, these members concentrated their comments on the publication record of the principal and co-investigators, the budget, and study design issues.

Discussions About the Principal Investigator

Many factors were discussed before scoring was performed. The track record of the principal investigator was of particular importance. Had they been funded in the past? Did they have a good publication record from their previous grants? Was their career productive, with multiple publications every year for the past five years, including first and senior author publications? Original research published by the investigator in high-impact journals as first or senior author was considered favorable. Case reports and review articles were not considered when assessing the number of publications. If a principal investigator presented a submission that was scientifically reasonable, but the individual had no first or senior author publications over the preceding five years, this was considered unfavorably. Even when the investigator had multiple publications over the previous five years, if they were purely multi-author publications and the investigator was not first or senior author, this suggested that the individual did not have the necessary profile to be a principal investigator.

The grant history of the principal investigator was also examined. If the principal investigator currently held two or more grants from the funding agency, the committee was less enthusiastic about providing an additional grant due to the questionable feasibility of successfully carrying out so many projects at once. On the other hand, being the recipient of few grants was also not viewed favorably. If the investigator included a reason for low productivity such as a maternity leave or health problems, this was taken into account.

Response to Previous Reviews

An important part of the committee's discussion revolved around the applicant's response to comments from previous reviewers. If the grant had been previously submitted and rejected, the investigator was given the opportunity to provide a two-page response to previous reviews. This response was particularly important, because the previous submission had been reviewed by the same committee, including some of the current committee members. If the application was re-submitted with few changes and no substantive responses to previous reviewer comments, it was not looked upon favorably.

Scoring

At this agency, grant applications are scored on a scale of 0–4.5. At the meeting I am describing, very few grants scored higher than 4.0. Those with a score greater than 4.0 were virtually assured of being funded, while grants with a score of less than 3.5 were clearly not going to be funded. During our meeting, no applications received a score of 4.4 or 4.5. Similarly, few applications scored below 3.0.

We applied a triage system when evaluating the grants. When the mean score of the first and second reviewers was less than 3.5, the grant was triaged without any discussion by the committee. The grant was not going to be funded. The investigators were subsequently provided with a rejection notification as well as detailed reviews from the first and second reviewers. If the average preliminary score of the first and second reviewers was greater than or equal to 3.5, then the committee proceeded to further discussion of the grant proposal.

Following discussion of the scientific value of the grant, the Chair determined a consensus score that could vary from the original scores awarded by the reviewers. Subsequently, each committee member individually scored the grant. We were able to score the grant 0.5 above or below the consensus score. For example, when the consensus score was 3.9, a committee member might personally score the grant from 3.4 to 4.4. Between 20 and 30% of all the grants submitted were triaged without discussion. It is important to note that the final scores from the committee did not exactly determine which grants received funding. Each funding agency has many grant review sub-committees. Each committee scores and ranks grant applications individually. Subsequently, grant scores are normalized across committees so that a similar percentage of grants are funded by each committee.

Certain issues decreased the scores of individual applications. For example, there was one grant in which half the grant consisted of plans for a clinical trial on humans, while the other half was an animal study. At the time, applicants were supposed to submit all randomized controlled trials to a particular committee at the funding agency. In this case, the investigators had violated the funding agency's rules by submitting a randomized controlled trial to a committee that was not equipped to review clinical trials. The committee recommended that the investigators separate the two components of the study and re-submit to the appropriate committees.

When reviewing another application, one of the reviewers printed out the publications by the principal investigator and noted that there appeared to be duplication of results in two of the papers. The committee considered this matter serious, and after discussing it at length, referred it to the ethics committee of the funding agency. That issue substantially decreased the score of the application, placing it in the non-fundable range.

Conflicts of Interest

Members of the committee who had a conflict of interest with an application stepped out of the room before the committee discussed it. Examples of conflicts of interest that precluded the participation of a committee member in the discussion included being friends with the principal investigator, having trained with the investigator, and having a close collaboration with the investigator. In the case of an investigator who worked at the same institution as the committee member, the committee member could still review the application and participate in the committee discussion, as long as they felt there was no conflict of interest. Before the committee discussions, committee members disclosed all potential conflicts of interest.

Tips for a Strong Grant Proposal

Below are some tips for writing a strong grant proposal that I learned while serving on various grant review committees (see Table 13.1 for additional tips).

1. The title of the grant application should be succinct and descriptive.

The title of your application should indicate the general purpose of your study. The committee members review many grants, so it is important to make yours easily recognizable. If you are submitting a systematic review or a meta-analysis, include this information in the title along with the topic (e.g., "A systematic review of five popular diets with respect to cardiovascular risk factors"). If you are submitting a

Table 13.1 Insider tips on the grant review process

1. Check what types of studies were previously funded by your target committee and for what amounts
2. "Fishing expeditions", even when well designed, are not viewed favorably
3. Conducting the same set of studies on a different group of patients is not viewed favorably
4. Small, prospective studies that are novel or hypothesis-generating do well
5. If you study an unfamiliar area, one of your co-investigators must be an established researcher in that area
6. Keep it simple and realistic
7. Avoid having too many hypotheses or separate experiments
8. Methodology is reviewed more rigorously in trials than in mechanistic studies
9. Emphasize science and biological/physiological mechanisms
10. If you include limitations, discuss in detail how you will deal with them
11. Discussion of study feasibility is important
12. Including preliminary pilot study data shows commitment, feasibility, and effect size for sample size calculations
13. Letters of collaboration are very important
14. Budget is of less significance than the proposal
15. Most committee members are content-oriented rather than methodologists
16. Remember that sample size estimates may be replicated by a committee member during the review
17. Even if most reviewers rate an application highly, the proposal can still be rejected based on relevance, feasibility, originality, and perceived ability of the investigators to do the job

randomized controlled trial, include an acronym for the study name (e.g., "Zyban as an Effective Smoking Cessation Aid: The ZESCA Trial"). If the grant is a renewal application, the title should be different from the title of the earlier submission. It is confusing to the committee when the investigator has several different grants with similar titles. Similar titles also raise the issue of how much overlap there is between the studies. As a result, each grant title should be distinctive. Because committees fund renewals at a much higher rate than de novo applications, the title should reflect the renewal status of the grant application.

2. The proposed duration should reflect the amount of work required.

From your point of view, it is preferable for the duration of funding to be as long as possible. The maximum duration allowed varies between funding agencies. The advantage of a longer duration is that you will not need to be constantly submitting grant applications in order to maintain funding. However, do not request an extended duration for a project that can be completed in a shorter amount of time. Committee members do not like this and will usually cut the duration; they may even reject the grant on this basis.

3. Spend time on the one-page summary.

Your one-page summary should be a succinct description of the rationale, methods, sample size calculations, expected results, and significance of your proposal.

Most committee members receive and read the full grant proposals only for the applications that are specifically assigned to them. As a result, your one-page summary might be the only document that they review during the committee meeting. For this reason, your summary should explain all elements that are important to a reader's understanding of your project and should be easily understood by individuals who are not content experts in that area. Many of the first and second reviewers who will review your application in detail will examine some sections very quickly. Your one-page summary is crucial to their understanding of your overall plans and to the likelihood of your grant being funded.

4. The lay summary of the grant should be clear and concise.

Some funding agencies ask for a lay summary. The lay summary is a single paragraph describing the grant application in layman's terms. This summary is useful to members of the committee who are not content experts in that area. In addition, if the funding agency decides that there needs to be a press release about the grant award at some point in the future, they may use your lay summary.

5. Clearly identify your study design.

In the one-page summary and study design sections, clearly describe your study design. For example, are you proposing a nested case control study, a cohort study, a randomized controlled trial, or a quasi-experimental design?

6. Provide accurate sample size and power calculations and clear plans for analyses.

The sample size calculations for each experiment should be clearly defined. If the sample size is based on the primary endpoint, then power calculations should be presented to show that the sample size would be adequate to examine the secondary and tertiary endpoints as well. In one of the review committee meetings I attended, there was an epidemiologist who came with his laptop and replicated the sample size and power calculations for each grant. You do not want to be in a position where you have an excellent research question and a well-written grant, only to discover that the committee is hesitant to recommend funding of your proposal because there is no evidence for choosing a particular sample size. Have a biostatistician involved in the grant process from the start who can provide you with well-conducted calculations. Similarly, your plans for data analysis need to be clear. Discuss which statistical analyses you will use, why, and how you will perform them. If you are not comfortable performing these types of analyses, then include a co-investigator who is a biostatistician and who will be able to perform them for you.

7. Outcomes should be "hard" and preferably "gold standard".

Grant review committees may love your proposed area of research but reject your application because of the particular outcomes you choose to study. Most biomedical sciences are quantitative. Because of this, "hard" outcomes are preferred. Hard outcomes are measurable events that are easy to quantify; they are not subjective. For example, number of deaths or myocardial infarctions are hard outcomes but angina is not. Often, there are many ways of measuring a given effect or event. The "gold standard" measure is the one that is widely accepted as being the best measure for a given outcome. If there is a viable hard outcome but you choose something less quantifiable and measurable, the committee will likely reject your application. If your outcome is the presence or absence of coronary disease, for example, it is not be ideal to use results of exercise stress testing as your outcome measure. Instead, committee members want to see hard, gold standard measures such as angiography, quantitative angiography, or intravascular ultrasound. The more well validated and harder your outcome, the more likely the committee will be in favor of your application. Sometimes, such measures are prohibitive because of the costs or the large number of patients required, or some other factor. If feasibility or cost is an issue, a committee may accept a surrogate measure, but you will need to justify your choice and explain how and why the substitute measure will be acceptable for your study.

8. Ensure that the research proposal is focused and easy to follow.

No two investigators write their research proposals in the same way. However, certain patterns emerge. For clinical research studies in which one major project is described, the first 40–50% of the proposal is usually dedicated to background and the remainder to study design. For basic science applications, there are usually multiple experiments proposed. For each experiment, include a background section followed by the study design. Each experiment builds on the previous experiment. Usually, there are three or more sequential experiments. For clinical research proposals, the first page of the grant application may be a recap of the one-page summary. This should be followed by the background section, which should read like a systematic review of the literature on this topic. For the funding agency I described earlier, the research proposal is 11–13 single-spaced pages in length, depending on the number of investigators involved in the application. The maximum allowable space should always be used. It does not reflect well on your proposal when there is more than one-quarter of a page left blank. Experienced investigators rarely leave blank spaces in grant applications.

9. Address the potential limitations of your grant.

Some investigators include a limitations section in their grants and others do not. If you do not have a limitations section, the reviewers will still identify the faults in your proposal, but you will not have the opportunity to refute them. In my opinion, you should always identify potential limitations and provide information in your proposal to persuade reviewers that they are not major limitations or that you can overcome or compensate for them. One way of doing this is to have a formal limitations section towards the end of your proposal. In that section, identify several potential limitations. Discuss how you will deal with them or why they are not true limitations. It is definitely not a good idea to identify limitations and not refute them.

10. Include pilot study data if possible.

Including pilot study data in an application is very helpful, even if they are preliminary. Grant review committees love to see pilot study data. The presence of pilot study in an application demonstrates that the principal investigator has been thinking about this problem for a while. It indicates that the investigator is committed to this area and has started researching it even though they have not yet been funded. Pilot study can provide you and the committee with practical information about the feasibility of the study. It can allow you to test case report forms and help you generate sample size data and power calculations. If possible, include a paragraph about pilot study data in your grant application and tables with pilot study in your appendices.

11. Include a strong CV module.

The committee wants to see that you have the experience, knowledge, and qualifications to successfully complete your proposed project. The CV module you include in your grant application is your chance to show that you have published results of previous studies and are capable of completing the proposed work.

Funding institutions have different requirements for the content and format of CVs. I describe the requirements for CVs at the agency where I reviewed to give you an idea of what should be included. The CV that accompanies a grant proposal at this funding agency consists of various sections. It begins with your current professional standing at your institution. For example, are you an assistant, an associate, or a full professor? Are you a section head, a division director, or a department head? This is followed by the "Funds Requested" section, which describes any grants or awards you have recently applied for. In this section, detail all applications you have submitted to funding agencies. This section is important, because the committee wants to know whether your grant application might be funded by another agency.

There is also a section entitled "Grants Held". This section informs the committee how many active grants you are currently involved in. If you are involved in multiple grants as a principal investigator, committee members may question whether you will have enough time to be involved in an additional major project. If you are involved in many different projects as a co-applicant, this is less of an issue. If you do not currently hold any operating grants, this may work for or against you. If the committee sees that there are gaps in your record during which you had no operating funds, they will question your productivity and your ability to maintain a research program. On the other hand, if this is your first application as a junior investigator or your first renewal, having few or no grants may work to your advantage because the committee will be reassured that you have the time to devote to this project.

In addition to a list of current grants, there is also a list of "Grants Held in the Past Five Years". This section documents recently completed grants. It provides committee members with an idea of how active you have been in the past five years, as well as the types of projects you were involved in, which agencies funded you, and how much funding they awarded to your projects.

You also have the opportunity to include supporting information about your career. In this section, detail your most important publications and explain why each contribution was important. This section also includes a record of your publications and abstracts over the previous five years. This section is crucial. The committee members will examine this section, particularly the publications, and decide whether you have been productive in terms of publishing in high-impact journals versus moderate- or low-impact journals. Did you publish reviews and editorials or original research? Did you consistently publish a minimum of two articles per year? Were there years when you did not publish any articles? Were you consistently the first or senior author? If you had multiple publications but were always in the middle of the author list, this will not be favorable. The committee does not closely examine abstracts; they will focus more on your publications and grants. Finally, include details about invited presentations and any patents you have acquired.

12. Append your prior publications.

There is often a section of the application where you can append some of your prior publications. These appended publications do not have to be in the same research area as your research proposal. Rather, the publications can demonstrate your productivity. Original first or senior author research articles published in high-impact journals are of value and should be appended, while review articles or editorials should not unless they are directly related to your research proposal. Appended publications should convince the committee members that you and your co-investigators are solid researchers with the ability to perform the proposed study.

13. Closely examine results of an unsuccessful submission before spending time revising it.

Take the notes from the Scientific Officer and the comments from the reviewers very seriously. These individuals have spent hours reviewing your proposal and their comments need to be addressed if you want to get the grant funded in the next competition. In particular, you need to read between the lines when examining the Scientific Officer's notes. Often, your score may be in the "good" but "not fundable" range. This might suggest that, with some additional tweaking, your application might reach the "fundable" range. However, close examination of the Scientific Officer's notes may indicate that none of the reviewers felt that the topic was particularly compelling. As a result, your grant may never become fundable, no matter how many adjustments you make to it. Consequently, it is extremely important that you closely examine the comments made by the Scientific Officer and the reviewers.

14. Include letters of collaboration.

Letters of collaboration are very important when submitting a grant proposal. A collaborator might perform the genetic analyses of the blood you collect or enroll patients in your clinical trial. Collaborators will help your project move forward but do not have the status of co-investigators. For your application, you will need letters from the individuals who will be collaborating on your study printed on their letterhead. They need to demonstrate enthusiasm and understanding of the project, and readiness to dedicate time and effort to accomplishing its objectives. Ideally, your collaborators will be individuals with significant past research experience. The inclusion of letters of collaboration from diversely talented individuals who are committed and enthusiastic is a major plus for any grant application. Make sure these letters say more than just how important your topic is; they should demonstrate practical commitments to the project and provide information that improves the feasibility of your project.

Summary

Before you embark on a new grant proposal, consult a more experienced colleague about your research project. Review several successfully funded grants before you put together your own. In addition, volunteer to review grants for a funding agency as either an external reviewer or internal reviewer. Serving as an internal committee member is an invaluable experience for a junior faculty member. It provides you with excellent insight into the grant review process and the components of a successful grant. Early exposure to the grant review process combined with guidance from experienced colleagues will significantly increase your chances of putting together a successful grant application.

Key Points

- First and second reviewers and the reader will provide detailed reviews of your application at the meeting before the committee discusses your proposal.
- Anyone who has a conflict of interest with members of a given research team is not allowed to be present when the grant proposal is being discussed.
- Each grant is given a score by committee members.
- Grants are funded in descending order of score.
- Provide a strong, comprehensive one-page summary; it may be the only document some of the reviewers read.
- Provide accurate sample size and power calculations and clear plans for analyses.
- Make it clear why your team is well suited to perform this research project.
- Address potential limitations.
- Thoroughly address comments from previous reviews in your response.
- Ensure that your CV and those of your co-investigators are strong and up-to-date.

Suggested Readings

1. Burroughs Wellcome Fund and Howard Hughes Medical Institute. Making the Right Moves: A Practical Guide to Scientific Management for Postdocs and New Faculty. 2nd ed. Research Triangle Park, NC; Chevy Chase, MD: Burroughs Wellcome Fund; Howard Hughes Medical Institute; 2006.
2. Sekikawa A, Aaron DJ, Acosta B, Nishimura R, LaPorte RE. Peer review of grant applications. Lancet 1998; 352: 1064.
3. Wessely S. Peer review of grant applications: what do we know? Lancet 1998; 352: 301–305.
4. Wingate CL. NIH peer review of grant applications. Definitions, procedures, and suggestions. Invest Radiol 1993; 28 (Suppl 2): S38–S40.

Chapter 14
Managing Your Team, Time, and Money

Management is doing things right. Leadership is doing the right things.

–Peter F. Drucker

Introduction

In this chapter, I discuss issues related to managing your research team, managing your time, and managing your research funds. Most new physician-scientists have limited training with respect to management issues. However, these issues are critical to your success as a physician-scientist. You may be an excellent physician and an excellent scientist, but unless you become adept at managing your research team, your time, and your research funds, you will have difficulty becoming optimally effective as a physician-scientist.

Managing Your Team

Creating and managing a research team is one of the most difficult tasks you will face as a new physician-scientist. You have probably been a member of several different research teams during your training as a physician-scientist. Although you performed your own projects as a member of these teams, you likely had little experience supervising laboratory technicians, research assistants, and students. Even though it is possible to succeed as a physician-scientist without a research team, it is unusual. Because of the limited time that physician-scientists have for research, they virtually always need a research team to maximize productivity. You will quickly find that if you work alone, you will be able to produce only one or two papers per year. If you have a well-functioning research team, you will be able to leverage your knowledge and skills into a much higher level of productivity. Although most beginning physician-scientists believe they should be in their offices working on papers, your primary role is to manage your research team.

M.J. Eisenberg, *The Physician Scientist's Career Guide*,
DOI 10.1007/978-1-60327-908-6_14, © Springer Science+Business Media, LLC 2011

Make-up of a Good Research Team

A good team equals more than the sum of the contributions of the individual members. A good team is synergistic; each member of the team brings something different to the table, so that the team as a whole is much more productive than the individual members working separately. As a physician-scientist, make sure you have substantive knowledge in your clinical area, as well as insight regarding the compelling questions you are researching. You should also be knowledgeable about different research techniques and procedures. You will have limited time to actually perform experiments yourself.

As I discussed in Chapter 8, you will be much more productive if you have a laboratory technician or research assistant to perform experiments under your supervision. You can also be more productive if you have a secretary who can help you prepare your manuscripts and grant applications. Summer students and graduate students can also be valuable additions to your team, and they can gain important experience while working with you. You should have a part-time financial officer on your team who can help you manage your budgets and grants. If you are conducting multi-center trials or clinical studies involving different sites, a research coordinator will be very beneficial. A biostatistician is critical and will help you with both the design and analysis of your projects. You will need to work with co-investigators and collaborators. Although you may have specific knowledge in one or two areas, having other team members with complementary skills and knowledge is a major plus. A multidisciplinary team, where each person brings something different to the table, will help you produce better quality research and a higher level of productivity than you would achieve on your own.

Assembling a Research Team

Assembling and managing a multidisciplinary research team is not a skill that most new physician-scientists are familiar with. As a new physician-scientist, this is one of the critical skills you will need to master early on or your career will flounder very quickly. Most physician-scientists have little or no experience with interviewing, hiring, conducting meetings, supervising students and research assistants, interacting with co-investigators, managing budgets, or balancing multiple projects at the same time.

Hiring

At the beginning of your career, you will usually have limited funds available to hire staff. I was in that situation. I did not know how to negotiate or obtain start-up funds when I interviewed for my first job. As a result, when I arrived at McGill as a new assistant professor, I had no money to hire staff. Fortunately, I received an e-mail within several weeks of my arrival indicating that new investigators could apply to have one or two summer students work for them for free. A government grant was available to pay the salaries of summer students interested in careers in healthcare. As a result, I began my research career with two undergraduate students. They had no previous research experience. Nevertheless, under my supervision, they were able to perform literature searches, copy articles, collect limited data, enter data, and create tables and figures. Because I provided them with an interesting research experience over the summer, they decided to continue working with me part-time as volunteers over the course of the year. Therefore, even if you have no resources whatsoever, you may be able to attract team members to help you perform your research, if you can offer them an interesting and beneficial experience. Potential sources include high school students, undergraduates, medical students, residents, fellows, and graduate students. Many of these individuals will be willing to help you with your research projects in exchange for research experience.

Finding Team Members

How do you find these individuals? At my institution, the research institute often receives letters and CVs from high school students and undergraduates interested in doing research. If you are not on the e-mail list for your research institute, ask them to include you on the list. Indicate that you are interested in hearing about anyone who applies to do research. All universities have electronic job boards. Find the job board on the web and upload an advertisement for a volunteer in your laboratory. Many hospitals accept high school students as volunteers. Contact the volunteer department at your hospital and see if there are any young people who might be interested in doing research. During your clinical activities in the hospital, make contact with medical students, residents, and fellows who may be interested in doing a research project with you. Make sure that graduate students who are looking for thesis supervisors are aware of your presence.

Research Assistants

Many of my paid research assistants over the past 15 years were students who had just finished their undergraduate studies and were taking one or two years off before going to medical school. These individuals are often extremely intelligent, highly motivated, and are willing to work long hours at low wages. Because most of my students were interested in entering medical school, they were more interested in the quality of their research experience than in their salary. I cannot afford high salaries in my laboratory. However, I have never had a problem attracting highly intelligent and motivated research assistants to help me conduct my research. Besides getting good experience, they often shadow me in the hospital to get an idea of what a practicing physician's life is like. They observe me interacting with patients and balancing different responsibilities. I invite them to my house once or twice a year so they can see that I also have a family life. Although they do not get rich from doing research in my laboratory, they obtain a very good understanding of what the life of a physician-scientist is like.

Research Associates

In addition to recent university graduates, I usually employ several full-time research associates. Research associates often have Masters-level education in a scientific discipline. Occasionally, they are graduate students who work part-time in my laboratory. I cannot pay these individuals as much as I would like. They certainly would receive much more if they worked in industry. However, they want the knowledge and the collegiality afforded by an academic environment. Besides doing much of the work involved in hiring new individuals, my senior research associates often manage projects and take on much of the responsibility for grant applications. Some of them function as mid-level managers of my research team. Without them, I would not be able to maximize the productivity of my team.

Importantly, my senior research associates now do most of the work of hiring for me. They upload the advertisements for our job postings. I forward all the CVs I receive to them, and they check the references and identify promising candidates. They then conduct the initial screening interviews with the candidates. Only once they have identified a candidate who they think is highly intelligent and motivated and who they think will work well on our team do they ask me to interview the individual. As a result, many of the tasks related to hiring are taken off my shoulders.

Professionals

As you become a more senior physician-scientist, your research team will mature. It will likely grow, and you will have more funds available to hire more experienced and better paid staff. These individuals may include laboratory technicians, research nurses, post-doctoral students, study coordinators, etc. Recruiting the right individuals for these positions is important because they are likely to stay with you for many years; perhaps even your whole career. To identify potential candidates, prepare a short advertisement that can be circulated electronically by your research institute. At the same time, talk to staff in the other laboratories at your institution to see if they know of any individuals looking for jobs. Professionals command higher salaries than research assistants. Be very particular about ensuring that the individuals you hire have the right qualifications, knowledge, and skills to perform the tasks that you require. It is important that you hire some mid- and senior-level individuals. As your research group grows, you will not be able to supervise all aspects of your laboratory. It is very helpful to have some mid- and senior-level individuals who can help you supervise your team.

Interviewing

I had no experience with interviewing or hiring prior to becoming a physician-scientist. However, I have learned a few important points over the past 15 years. Number one is to be careful about whom you hire. It is much more difficult to end a working relationship than it is to start one. Most of the time, this is not a problem.

Occasionally, however, you will hire an individual who is problematic and who you wish you had never hired in the first place.

Before hiring anyone, I require a cover letter indicating their interest and background as well as a CV. If they have recently graduated, I also ask for transcripts. I always contact references. If I think that the individual may make a good addition to our research team, and if they pass the screening interviews with my senior research associates, I interview them myself. These interviews take place in my office and are relatively informal. I want to get an idea of whether this individual is someone who will fit into our research team. I assess whether they are intelligent, personable, engaging, motivated, and a team player. It is important to me that they have good writing skills. If I am unsure about this point, I will sometimes give them a writing exercise to complete. I also want to see that they have adequate skills with various computer programs.

I often recruit for particular positions. For example, for a research assistant who will be in contact with patients or with research nurses at other institutions, I want someone who is outgoing and personable. For a research assistant who will be doing a detailed literature review and data abstraction, I want someone who can remain focused for long periods of time. As a result, depending on the position, I look for a slightly different type of individual.

Some of the questions that I ask during an interview are as follows:

- Why do you want to work with our research group?
- What did my senior research associates explain to you about what we do in this research group?
- What are your long-term goals?
- How well do you work in groups?
- What are your writing skills like?
- How long can you commit to working with our team?
- Do you recognize that the salary is quite low?
- Do you have any background in statistics?

In addition to the questions above, I also try to get a feel from where this individual is coming. Where were they born? Where is their family? Are they planning on staying in the city for the foreseeable future? I spend lots of time with members of my research team. If I am put off by an individual during the interview, I have found that it is probably not a good idea to hire them. It is important that a research assistant can commit to working for me for at least 12 months. It often takes months before they understand all the ins and outs of my laboratory. It also takes months before they understand how I like to have my manuscripts and grant applications formatted, the way I like my presentations put together, etc. I do not want to hire and train a research assistant only to find that they will be leaving after a few months.

Typically, I hire research assistants in the spring. At a minimum, they need to commit to working the entire summer, the next academic year, and the following summer. The reason for this is that I need an overlap of one or two months between old and new research assistants. This usually occurs during the summer. This is when the new research assistants are trained by the old research assistants. If there is no overlap, then I will be the one responsible for training them. I need a solid research team during the summer when turnover occurs. Also, summers are the times when I have large numbers of students conducting research projects. These students need more supervision than I can provide alone. As a result, I need my more experienced research associates to be present during the summer.

Expanding Your Team

As the leader of a research team, you always need to be thinking one or two years ahead. What is the funding outlook for your group? What types of projects will you be involved in? Will some members of the team be leaving? As you become a more senior physician-scientist, you will likely accumulate more grant support and be involved in a growing number of projects of more ambitious scope. To perform these projects, your research team needs to grow accordingly. You will be hiring fewer junior research assistants and will need to hire professionals with particular skill sets for the long term. Be cognizant of this. Get the opinions of other members of your team and of senior physician-scientists. Think about the number and types of staff you will need and start the hiring process early. You do not want to be in a position where you receive substantial grant support but do not have sufficient staff to start a project.

Strategies for Managing Your Team

Some individuals are born with intrinsic management skills. Most of us are not. If you want to be successful at managing your research team, you need to develop management skills. Many of these skills are things you learned when you were young. Do not give orders. Be polite. Share your time with others. Share your skills and knowledge. Be pleasant. Inquire about the welfare of others. Make sure you are approachable. Make sure you have time for each individual on your team. Effective management of your research team is critical to your scientific success. Without skilled management of your team, your research career will not succeed. Your team needs guidance so that everyone is going in the same direction. You need to provide the motivation for the team. There are several strategies I have found that help me manage my team.

Individual Meetings

Meet with each member of your team individually on a regular basis. Ideally, this should occur at least once a week for 20–30 minutes. Spend most of this time discussing their individual projects. They might show you some of their initial results; you might discuss some of the problems they are having with their projects; or they might show you a draft of their manuscript. A beginning research assistant or student will occasionally go off on a tangent if not supervised closely. As a result, particularly at the beginning of your relationship, it is a good idea to have regular contact to make sure that you are both on the same page. During these meetings, it is important to ask how they are doing. What are their plans for the future? Be sincerely interested in the welfare of your research assistants and students. Their success is your success.

Small Group Meetings

In addition to individual meetings, I meet on a regular basis with small groups within my research team. These groups are composed of individuals involved in particular projects. For example, if my team is composed of ten members, two or three of them may be working on a particular project. I meet with these individuals to see how that particular project is progressing. Often, the project members will approach me and request to meet about a particular issue. For this reason, I try to keep my door open and be available during the day for discussions with team members.

Business Meetings

In a large research team, many members may not know what other members of the team are doing. For this reason, I hold a business meeting approximately once a month. I find it helpful to have a prearranged agenda for the meeting. The agenda helps ensure that we discuss every ongoing project. In addition, it helps us review the different responsibilities of each individual in the group. During the meeting, we do not discuss a lot of the details about the individual projects. Rather, we summarize what the projects are about, how they are progressing, and what are the expected timelines. Here are some typical questions that we discuss during a business meeting:

- When is the grant submission deadline?
- When is the paper expected to be submitted for publication?
- Are there any major problems so far?
- Will any members of the team be absent? If so, when and for how long?
- Do we need additional computers prior to the arrival of the summer students?
- Do we have sufficient printers? What about toner?
- Is there additional software that needs to be purchased?
- What abstracts are going to be submitted for the next deadline?
- When are the next scientific meetings taking place?
- Who will be attending?

I also address security issues during business meetings. I am particularly concerned about the security of our computer network. I remind individuals to keep their doors locked and their personal items secure. The final item on the agenda is always when will the next social event take place? By having an official business meeting approximately once a month, we ensure that every individual in the group knows what their responsibilities are and what the other members of the team are doing.

Research Meetings

We try to hold research meetings once a week, particularly during the summer when large numbers of students are present. These meetings are different from business meetings and consist of the presentation of research in progress. Individual team members present a particular project in detail. They have 30–45 minutes to describe their project. If their project is in its early stages, they might describe the background and the methodology. If the project is almost completed, they might present some of the results and discuss what they mean. It is important for students and research assistants to have the opportunity to present their results in an informal setting and receive informal feedback. Many of these sessions include practice presentations prior to presentations at major conferences.

Steering Committee Meetings

Several other activities can be used to promote team cohesion and to show team members that you value them. One activity is the inclusion of team members in meetings with co-investigators of various collaborative projects. For example, I am the principal investigator for several multi-center clinical trials. During steering committee meetings with co-investigators, I always include the students and research assistants who are involved in the project. In addition to observing the discussion, I also give them the occasional opportunity to speak to the steering committee about a particular aspect of the project. This demonstrates that I value their experience and contributions to the project. Frequently, the research assistant has much more insight into a particular aspect of the study than the principal investigator and the co-investigators.

Division Meetings

My research group is located within the Division of Clinical Epidemiology at my hospital. The division hosts its own conferences, in addition to those arranged by our research team. I encourage every member of my group to attend the weekly epidemiology seminar held by the division. Besides learning about projects taking place outside our research group, it also gives members of my team the opportunity to interact with members of other laboratories within our division. The principal investigators of the different laboratories, their senior research associates, and their graduate students often present at these meetings. These meetings give the members of my laboratory the opportunity to gain some academic exposure to the wider area of clinical epidemiology. These interactions are important from a scientific point of view, and they also help foster a collegial environment.

Research Day

I try to send my research assistants and students to present at student research days and to submit abstracts to national and international meetings. This greatly benefits the team members, because it gives them valuable practice in describing their work to others. The ability to present research in a clear and interesting manner to both experts and non-experts in your field is an essential skill for a physician-scientist. If at all possible, try to attend their presentations. Not only does this demonstrate that you believe their presentation is important, but also provides you with a very good idea about their understanding of their research project.

Conferences, Meetings, and Courses

Encourage your team members to attend conferences, meetings, and courses. Although it is expensive and time-consuming to send your team members out of town, it sends an important message to them. It shows that you are interested in their welfare, in advancing their education, and that you think they are important members of your laboratory. Because team members are often paid low salaries, this is one of the perks you can give them to keep them motivated. It also helps your research program, because members come back with new insights into their own research projects as well as ideas for new projects. They also represent your laboratory at national and international meetings, which shows that your team continues to be productive. Thus, you should encourage them to attend meetings and conferences regularly. I also try to send them to courses to learn skills such as how to coordinate a multi-center trial.

Annual Planning Meeting

Approximately once a year, I meet with individual members of my team to review their plans for the future. For Master's students, I ask them whether they will be pursuing a PhD. If they are a PhD student, I want to know what they are planning to do next. Will they go into academia or industry? Will they leave the city for post-doctoral training? How is their spouse handling their graduate studies? If they are an undergraduate, are they planning on pursuing graduate studies? Are they planning on applying to medical school? What is their timeline? This meeting offers team members the opportunity to seek career advice. Not only does it demonstrate that you are interested in them as individuals, it also helps you gauge how many members of your laboratory will be present over the next year or two. Without this knowledge, it is difficult to plan the logistics of your future projects. This is a mutually beneficial process and an important part of mentoring your team and managing your laboratory.

Social Events

In addition to team meetings, it is important to have regular social events. Once or twice a year, I invite my research team to my house for dinner. Following dinner, we often have a movie night where we watch a movie projected on a wall in my basement while eating popcorn. On other occasions, we go out for dinner or play a sport. We regularly go out for sushi. We occasionally play basketball, hockey, or soccer. My family often joins us during these events. I receive a lot of positive feedback from my research team about these social events. They particularly enjoy coming to my house and meeting my wife and children and realizing that I have a life outside of the hospital.

Another event that I hold is the annual "junk food lunch". This has been a tradition in my laboratory since I first became an assistant professor. The "junk food lunch" involves sending members of the group to a local supermarket to buy only junk food for lunch. I have them buy food that is as artificial in color or appearance as possible. Although I recognize that this is not a healthy practice, it is an event that everyone looks forward to and is discussed by the group for months in advance and months afterwards. It is a signature event every summer and is almost a rite of initiation in my laboratory.

In addition to social events in which the entire group participates, it is not unusual for individual members or for the whole group to get together without me. I think that this is very healthy. Many previous members of my research team have remained close friends. Two of them even married and are now parents. It is important for every research group to have occasional social activities. It gives the group a sense of solidarity. We are not just co-workers; we are members of a team.

Planning for Departures

Virtually all team members eventually leave your laboratory. You need to recognize that this is going to happen. Hopefully, you will be aware of all departures well in advance. If an individual is a key research assistant or technician, make sure that you hire someone with similar skills in advance of their departure. You need at least one month of overlap between the old staff member and the new one in order for key skills and knowledge to be passed on. New team members, whether a student or a research assistant, need to have an idea of the different projects that are going on in your laboratory. It can be very disruptive to the balance of a laboratory when key members leave and new members are not in place to take over their responsibilities. Plan ahead and make sure that there is significant overlap between members who are leaving and members who are arriving. You cannot have a research coordinator for a large multi-center clinical trial leave the laboratory and have a new coordinator start 1 week later. There is much unwritten information that needs to be transferred between the two individuals. You can minimize this issue by having your employees keep detailed records of how they perform their tasks. For example, maintain files of important websites and contact information to pass on to new employees. Also keep any documents pertaining to current manuscripts and grants on file for reference. Keep templates for letters, papers, and other documents to minimize the amount of work that must be redone each time a particular task needs to be repeated. However, even if you carefully document as many tasks as possible, there will be a lot of information that your old assistant will need to explain to his or her replacement.

Letting Someone Go

Occasionally, you will need to let someone go from your laboratory. This can be an extremely difficult experience, particularly when you are a new physician-scientist and have not done it before. There can be various reasons for having to let someone go, including a personality conflict, a lapse of ethics, a lack of motivation and productivity, or a lack of team spirit. Whatever the reason, it is important that you do not create undue animosity when you let this person go. Importantly, ensure that this individual does not sabotage any projects when they leave. If you think that this is a possibility, make sure that you let them go on a Friday afternoon. Then, change all the passwords on the computers and terminate this individual's access to your laboratory. In addition, all members of your laboratory need to be aware that this person has been let go and that they should not release any confidential information to them. In a case where you anticipate that you will have to let someone go, prepare a personnel file in advance. Record any lapses that occurred at the time they occur. These lapses should be discussed with the individual when they occur. Make it clear to them that, if these lapses continue, you will be forced to let them go. It is clearly not optimal to let someone go without prior warning.

Managing Your Time

One of the most important determinants of whether you will be a successful physician-scientist is how you manage your time. When you are a beginning physician-scientist, there are many responsibilities that require your attention. These responsibilities include teaching, administration, research, clinical responsibilities, and family activities. Because of these competing responsibilities, it is important that you use your time efficiently. Maximize and concentrate the amount of time available for you to do research. It is not a good idea to have one hour at a time for research, separated by other responsibilities. You need long periods of time in which you can focus on your research program.

The amount of time you have for protected research is critical. If you have 80% of your time protected for research, you theoretically have four of the five working days per week to do research. However, this does not take into account your on-call availability during nights and weekends or time away for conferences and vacations. You will also need time for administrative activities, committee meetings, teaching activities, etc. Therefore, it is very important at the beginning of your career to form a strong research team that can function when you are absent doing your other activities. At the same time, be very disciplined about managing your time so that you can be maximally productive.

You should have a strong research foundation with a well-funded program and many projects in different stages of progression. Be constantly thinking about new ideas for projects. You should have projects that are just starting, projects that are midway through, and projects that are nearing completion; this will create a strong research pipeline. As a junior physician-scientist, it is important to have multiple research projects. Some should be short term and some should be long term. Short-term projects will help maintain your productivity while you are conducting long-term ones. Some of your projects will be "long shots" and others will be "sure things." You need to take some risks, but not too many. You can take more risks as you get further along in your career. Demonstrate productivity and an ability to attract funding at the beginning of your career. Only once you obtain tenure and are an established researcher should you pursue risky long-term projects that might not bear fruit. One of the keys to good time management is to divide your time between each of your projects. If you spend all your time focused on the project with the nearest deadline, you will not be able to accomplish the ambitious projects on your agenda that take months and years to accomplish.

Delegating and Leveraging

Because each of us has a limited amount of time protected for research, it is important to manage our time carefully. For this reason, delegate as many activities as possible so that you are able to leverage your time. Delegating activities does not come naturally to most new physician-scientists. This might be the first time that you have had a secretary or a research assistant. Nevertheless, you need to quickly identify and delegate activities that can be done by someone else. Your time should be reserved for doing activities that only you can perform. As a result, activities like writing business letters, sending reprints, setting up databases, entering data, doing literature searches, and printing out PDFs should all be delegated. Your time should be reserved for identifying new projects, writing papers, performing revisions of grant proposals, preparing revisions of papers that are provisionally accepted at journals, and activities of a similar nature.

Most individuals can write only a handful of first author papers per year. With all your other responsibilities, you will have limited time to write papers. However, if you develop a research team with individuals of different strengths and abilities, you will become more productive with little additional effort. A secretary who is experienced at writing business letters and formatting grant proposals and papers can save you a lot of time. Similarly, a research coordinator who can manage a project once it is in place is also a great time saver. A research coordinator can coordinate a large multi-center clinical trial, in which patients are being enrolled at many different clinical sites, with fairly limited input from you. Meet with your coordinator once a week and get an update on the issues. Become involved only when there is an issue that needs a top-level decision. Similarly, you can have multiple medical students, residents, and fellows working simultaneously on different projects. They will largely work independently, and you may only need to meet with them once every week or two depending on the project. In this way, you can be involved in many different studies that are moving forward at a fast pace without doing all the legwork. Reserve your time for supervising the projects and addressing the major problems that arise.

Ideally, you should train a laboratory supervisor who can run much of the day-to-day activity of your laboratory. For example, if you have a graduate or post-doctoral student who has proven that they can be a good manager, this individual should supervise many of your other team members. They can potentially write first drafts of some grant proposals. They can manage some projects, with your involvement being required only when major questions arise. Most productive laboratories have many individuals involved, and it can be difficult for a busy physician-scientist to closely supervise each of them. As a result, it is essential that you recruit a laboratory supervisor who will run the day-to-day activities. In this way, your time can be freed up for more strategic activities such as identifying new areas of research, identifying new topics for grant proposals, and being closely involved in the writing and submission of manuscripts.

It is easy to get involved in peripheral activities. For example, you can get bogged down responding to e-mails and surfing the Web. These activities may be tangentially related to your research but are not high value-added activities. Develop a schedule with fixed times when you commit to doing high-yield activities, like writing and revising papers and grant proposals. These times should be free of competing activities, such as phone calls or meetings with medical students, residents, fellows, or research assistants. It is not uncommon for physician-scientists to say, after several years of their career, that they have no time left to do research or to write papers. If this is your case, it is because you are not managing your time well and are not delegating activities in a way that allows you to be optimally productive.

Managing Your Research Funds

Besides managing your research team and your time, you need to develop expertise at managing your research funds. Most junior physician-scientists have little experience managing large quantities of money. This is an important topic and one that you need to quickly become familiar with. If you ignore this issue, you could get into trouble. Be aware of what you can and cannot use your grant support for, how to put together a budget, and what the differences are when budgeting for peer-reviewed and industry-sponsored grants.

Role of the Research Institute

At most academic medical centers, research funds are managed by the research institute. When you obtain an operating grant, the money goes to the research institute of your hospital. Although the funds are at your disposal to use for research purposes, you do not have direct access to these funds. An account is set up in the name of the project. To use the funds, you must submit invoices to the research institute (often using particular forms). Checks are then sent directly from the institute to the appropriate place. For example, if you are running a multi-center trial, each time you want to reimburse a particular site for the enrollment of patients, you are required to send an invoice to the institute with the date, the name of the institution, the address where the check should be sent, the amount, and the reason for the debit. Your institute and the granting agency might audit your accounts, so familiarize yourself with the rules specific to your institution and the granting agencies you deal with.

Role of the Financial Officer

Each research institute has a financial officer. This individual keeps track of the accounts of all researchers. They periodically provide statements for your accounts. It is important to review these statements when they come to you. You do not want to be in a position where you have not completed your research project but your funds have been completely depleted. Similarly, you do not want to come to the end of the project and find that you have a large balance in your account. If this occurs, the residual funds need to be returned to the funding agency that awarded the grant. Each institute has specific rules regarding the types of activities that can be reimbursed from your research accounts. Become familiar with these rules before you receive your first grant.

Direct Versus Indirect Costs

Research grants are composed of direct and indirect costs. Direct costs are those associated with paying staff (including benefits), buying equipment, paying for travel, etc. In the US, staff costs need to be justified according to percent effort, and investigator salaries are considered direct costs. In Canada, investigator salaries are covered by separate salary support grants. Indirect costs are those associated with non-tangible items like computer infrastructure, insurance, security, etc. If you are funded by the NIH, part of the budget is for direct costs and part is for indirect costs. Because you are probably not familiar with the indirect costs of your project, your research institute will help you prepare your budgets in this regard. In Canada, research institutes receive direct funding from funding agencies to cover indirect costs. Importantly, grants from industry are treated differently than grants from peer-reviewed funding agencies. In most institutions, a certain percentage of the budget from an industry-associated grant will be taken off the top for indirect costs. For example, if you receive an industry-related grant of $1 million, your institute may take 30% ($300,000) off the top, leaving you with only $700,000 to cover the direct costs of your project.

Managing Accounts

Most active researchers have multiple active accounts. If you have 10 funded projects, you will have 10 different accounts. Ensure that the invoices for a particular project are invoiced to the correct account and not to that of another project. As much as possible, try to adhere to the budget you submitted when your funding was approved. There is some latitude allowed here. For example, you may need to increase the number of sites that are recruiting for your study or the per-patient reimbursement. As long as you do not run a deficit, you will usually not be questioned about your expenses; nevertheless, be prepared to justify your expenses in case of an audit. In addition, remember that most funds from peer-reviewed agencies come from tax payers or charities, so you have an ethical responsibility to spend them wisely on the costs for which they were intended.

Expenses

Every institution has explicit guidelines about which expenses are valid and which are not. Familiarize yourself with these guidelines. For example, if you fly to a research meeting in another city, most institutions will not pay for first class seats. If you attend a research meeting and add on a few days of vacation, you can be reimbursed for the flights and the hotel accommodations incurred during the meeting, but you are responsible for the balance of the hotel accommodations. Most of these guidelines are intuitive, but it is useful to review and become familiar with them and with any unusual details. For example, your institution may pay a per diem for food so that you do not need to collect receipts. You will likely find that there is a fixed reimbursement for car travel depending on the distance. Your institution may also pay for certain expenses like registrations to meeting and flights in advance, so that you do not need to carry the balance on your credit card for an extended period of time. It is helpful to sit down with your financial officer and review all the details that are specific to your institution.

Start-Up Funds

A new physician-scientist is typically provided with some start-up funds. In the case of a physician-scientist with a basic science laboratory, these funds may be substantial. Funds are to be used to purchase the equipment and supplies that you will need to become successful in your research area. In the case of a physician-scientist who does not have a basic science laboratory, the amount of start-up funds may be much less. Whatever resources you have need to be used judiciously so that you have the best chance at succeeding in your career. When negotiating for your first job, be explicit in your request for start-up funds. Be realistic in terms of what you need. Beginning your career with no start-up funds could severely impede your ability to do research. At the very least, you will need funds to purchase a computer and software, to hire a half-time secretary and a part-time research assistant or laboratory technician, and to purchase the bare minimum of equipment needed to perform your research. If all your time during the first one or two years is spent writing grants to obtain funds so that you can do your research, your career will get off to a slow start and may even fail.

Financial Commitment to New Physician-Scientists

A new appointee will typically receive a guarantee of salary support, start-up funds, and protected time for research for the first three–five years. If you are not successful in obtaining an operating grant, producing some high-quality publications, and perhaps obtaining a career award during that period, your time will no longer be protected and you will usually be forced to switch to full-time clinical status. If you are able to obtain a five-year commitment to support your research, it will take a large weight off your shoulders. As a result, you will not be overly concerned if your grant applications are not funded during the first one or two cycles. That is not to say that you should not focus on obtaining grant support, but you will have a less pressured time frame in which to get your program off the ground.

Additional Funds for Junior Investigators

Internal funds are often available to junior investigators to begin pilot studies. The availability of these funds may not be widely known, so you need to inform yourself about them. Although these awards may not be large, they can make a big difference in getting your career off the ground. You can use this money to pay a research assistant or to perform a pilot study that could help you obtain a peer-reviewed operating grant. In addition, if you are successful at obtaining internal funds, it will look favorable on your applications to funding agencies for peer-reviewed grant support.

Summary

Managing your research team, your time, and your research funds can be major challenges for a new physician-scientist. If you are not experienced in management issues, you need to learn these skills quickly. Only through successful management of your team, your time, and your research funds can you be maximally productive. I urge you not to ignore these aspects of being a physician-scientist. It is critical to the success of your career.

Key Points

- Create a research team that is maximally productive.
- Delegate non-essential tasks so that you can reserve your time for high-value activities.

- An effective team is multidisciplinary; everyone brings a different skill.
- Research assistants need to commit to working for you for at least one year.
- Individual meetings, small group meetings, business meetings, research meetings, and social events are good ways to motivate your team.
- Review statements provided by your Financial Officer to ensure your budget is on track.
- Negotiate start-up funds so that you can hire assistants and begin your research ASAP.
- Check the availability of internal funds at your institution.

Suggested Readings

1. Getting Started: Team Meeting Tools. http://www.americanheart.org/presenter.jhtml?identifier =1882. Accessed May 11, 2009.
2. Andrade FH. Starting a new lab: developing new techniques and hiring personnel. Physiologist 2008; 51: 188–190.
3. Brooks RR. Management tips. Managing people, time, paperwork. AORN J 1988; 48: 1139–1143.
4. Dye CF. Hiring: get it right the first time. Healthc Financ Manage 2007; 61: 116–118.
5. The Clinician Scientist: Yesterday, Today and Tomorrow. http://www.cihr-irsc.gc.ca/e/ 12970.html. Accessed April 7, 2009.
6. Mohan-Ram V. Negotiating: please sir, can I have some more? Sci Career Mag 2000.
7. Nelson LE, Morrison-Beedy D. Research team training: moving beyond job descriptions. Appl Nurs Res 2008; 21: 159–164.
8. Silva TD, da Cunha Aguiar LC, Leta J, et al. Role of the undergraduate student research assistant in the new millennium. Cell Biol Educ 2004; 3: 235–240.
9. The Team Meeting. http://www.teambuildinginc.com/tps/020 g.htm. Accessed May 11, 2009.
10. Negotiating for What You Need to be Successful. http://serc.carleton.edu/NAGTWorkshops/ careerprep/jobsearch/negotiating.html. Accessed May 12, 2009.

Chapter 15
Mentorship

Mentor: someone whose hindsight can become your foresight.
–Unknown

Introduction

Navigating each stage of the physician-scientist career path is challenging. Because there is no blueprint for this pathway, it is sometimes difficult to know what is expected of you at each stage. Having good mentors throughout your career can help make the challenges more manageable. Finding the right mentor can be difficult. A mentor who is good at one stage of your career may not be the right mentor for you at another stage of your career. It can be difficult to know where to find mentors and how to approach them. In some institutions, new physician-scientists receive formal mentorship during the first few years of their career. This may also happen for individuals who are training as physician-scientists. However, in the majority of situations, formal mentorship is not offered. Instead, it is up to you to find mentors, to develop relationships with them, and to identify the help that you need from them. As you become more senior, it is your responsibility to serve as a mentor for younger individuals. This role may not be one for which you have had specific training. However, each of us has encountered different mentors along the physician-scientist pathway. Some have been good and others have not. By identifying the good and not so good qualities in our own mentors, we can develop the traits needed to be effective mentors ourselves.

My Experiences

Like all physician-scientists, I have encountered various mentors along my career pathway. Some have been excellent and others less so. Though I already discussed some of my own training experiences in Chapter 1, in this chapter, I describe in detail some of the traits of mentors that I have encountered and some of the lessons I learned from them about mentorship.

M.J. Eisenberg, *The Physician Scientist's Career Guide*,
DOI 10.1007/978-1-60327-908-6_15, © Springer Science+Business Media, LLC 2011

Undergraduate Research

As a university undergraduate, I performed research for several years in a bio-chemistry laboratory. My mentor was a new assistant professor who was trying to generate a track record in research in order to obtain tenure. His laboratory was small and did not involve many individuals. He was a very friendly and helpful individual, and I had a good relationship with him. Although my mentor had very good intentions, ultimately, my experience in his laboratory was not particularly fruitful. I spent several years working part time in the laboratory, but I did not have any publications to show for it at the end. A large part of this was because I was not a particularly good basic science researcher. My experience in this laboratory was intended to help me investigate whether I was interested in basic science research. In that sense, the experience was good, because I found that it was not satisfying. At the same time, however, I think that it would have been useful for my mentor to ensure that I was involved in at least one publication. One of the great pleasures of doing research is being involved in data analysis and manuscript writing. Without the positive feedback of a publication, a student may feel that they have not had a very successful experience. Also, I think that part of my problem was that I wanted to go to medical school, so a basic science biochemistry laboratory was not really in sync with my clinical interests. It is very important to make sure that your mentor's interests are in line with yours. When you are a mentor yourself, you need to recog-nize the type of mentee who will benefit from exposure to you. This issue needs to be evaluated carefully at the beginning of any mentor–mentee relationship.

Year Off During Medical School

I took a year off between my second and third year of medical school. During this period, I spent some time in another laboratory doing bench research. My experi-ence was not ideal. Although I was very interested in the research project, I had little access to my mentor. My role in the project was to help a technician analyze blood. This was a very repetitive technical job that did not engage me intellectually. Doing this job would have been all right if I had also been involved in some data analysis and writing. In addition, I wanted some exposure to the patients that we were study-ing, since my interests were both clinical and research-oriented. However, I had limited access to patients as well. Thus, this experience reinforced for me that I was not meant for basic science research. It also taught me about the type of mentor that I wanted to be. Being a good mentor means being accessible to your mentee. You cannot just accept someone as a mentee and then leave them with a technician and expect that they will have a satisfying and intellectually stimulating experience. Particularly for a student who is trying to gain career-related exposure, you need to provide a well-rounded experience. For a mentee to have a good research experi-ence, they need to be involved in several different aspects of the project. You have a responsibility to teach trainees multiple skills besides the technical aspects of your research. They need to get experience reviewing the literature, analyzing data, and writing. Most importantly, you need to be available, accessible, and enthusiastic.

Cardiology Elective in Medical School

As a fourth year student in medical school, I did a cardiology elective, which involved a month with a cardiologist who was a physician-scientist. I shadowed him in clinic, on rounds in the hospital, and during his interactions with patients. Although he was a physician-scientist, I did not have any interactions with him vis-a-vis his research. Nevertheless, my experience with him left me with a very favorable impression of how to be a physician-scientist. I knew that this individual produced well-respected research. He published influential articles on clinically important topics in high impact journals. At the same time, my day-to-day experiences with him showed me that he was an excellent clinician who truly cared for his patients. As part of this elective, he had me write a review article on a topic of my choice. This experience gave me an exciting opportunity to evaluate the literature in a particular area. I very much enjoyed this experience. My mentor reviewed the article once I had written it, and he gave me helpful comments. The manuscript became my first publication in the medical literature. When I mentor younger individuals, I try to emulate some of the traits that I saw in this individual. In particular, I try to allow my pre-medical and medical students to shadow me during cardiology consultations, in the cardiac catheterization laboratory, in the cardiac care unit, and in my clinic. Although these students are primarily involved with me for research, even a day or two of clinical exposure helps them to conceptualize the idea of a physician-scientist who balances both research and clinical work. Allowing them to see what I do clinically makes them much more likely to consider becoming physician-scientists.

Mentorship During Residency

When I was a first year resident in internal medicine, I developed a mentor who was a cardiologist and a physician-scientist. I came to this individual with a research project that I wanted to do, and he agreed to supervise me. He also wanted me to do one of his projects. He was very accessible and enthusiastic, making my research elective a very positive experience. He was an unconventional thinker. He was provocative and somewhat eccentric. However, he was the kind of person that I could relate to; his interests spanned the spectrum of clinical medicine and research. Not only did I get to be exposed to him clinically and research-wise, but he also invited me to his home and to his country house with his family. These social experiences helped to consolidate my relationship with him. The only aspect of this relationship that was less fruitful was the fact that at the end of my data collection for both projects, he was not able to help me analyze the data. My projects were more epidemiology-oriented, and he was more of a basic science researcher. Thus, I needed to be referred to outside people in order to complete the data analysis and write up the papers. This experience taught me that not all mentors can provide everything we need. Because each physician-scientist's career is unique, no single person can teach you all the knowledge and skills that you need.

Mentor at the Harvard School of Public Health

During my MPH, I did a tutorial course with an emeritus professor of epidemiology. I met with this individual once per week, and he helped me analyze the data from the two projects I performed during my residency. Each week, he reviewed my data and suggested new ways of analyzing it. With his help, I was able to write papers for the two projects from my residency that I had previously been unable to complete. From my point of view, it was a highly successful experience. Although this individual was not a physician-scientist, he was an expert with a skill set that I needed access to. Besides helping me with my data analysis, we had some interesting discussions about large clinical trials that he had been involved with. It was exciting to learn behind-the-scenes information about articles that I had read in high-impact journals. This experience showed me that you do not need to be able to mentor your mentee in all the skills they need. Sometimes you have a very particular expertise which you can expose the student to.

Research Experience After Residency

I took another year off after my internal medicine residency. During this time, I spent six months doing clinical research. My mentor had a particular research question that he wanted me to address using a previously developed database. Unfortunately, I was left largely on my own. Not only was I in an unfamiliar environment, but I also had very little research direction. I had limited access to this individual, and even when I did have access to him, he was not particularly helpful in terms of moving the project forward. Ultimately, I was able to analyze the data and write up a paper. However, I felt that I could have been much more productive with a more satisfactory mentor–mentee relationship. This experience drove home the message that it is not fair to accept responsibility to be a mentor and then not be accessible to the mentee. If you are going to accept the responsibility of being a mentor, you need to recognize that your mentee has certain needs which you have to be able to accommodate. Otherwise, the experience will not be productive for either one of you.

Finding Mentors: What to Look for

The type of mentor that you need varies depending on your stage in the physician-scientist pathway. When you are an undergraduate, you need a mentor who is able to explain things to you simply and who has time to spend with you. When you are a research trainee, you may require less direct contact with your mentor, but you still need someone who is empathetic, who understands what level you are at, and who will not begrudge their time to teach you the skills that you need. No matter what stage you are at, your mentor needs to be committed to mentoring and teaching research skills. Your mentor needs to have time to give you feedback on your presentations and papers and to guide you through the research and publication process. You need a person who is willing to sit down over a cup of coffee and give you some ideas about what trajectory your career might take.

The only way you can really identify such an individual is by talking to them. At each stage of your career, I would encourage you to identify several potential mentors and to talk with them informally about your situation. In some cases, such as when you are looking for a laboratory to do your research training, you are looking for a formal mentor. In other cases, such as when you are a new physician-scientist, you are looking for an informal mentor such as a mid-career or senior level investigator who will be able to help you through the grant application process. There are likely to be several candidates for such roles at your institution. You need to sit down with these individuals and discuss your situation. You will quickly see who has time to spend with you, who is willing to collaborate on projects, and who can spend time giving you feedback.

Mentors can provide useful advice on various topics. Because they have already gone through the system, they can share their wisdom with you. If you just sit in your laboratory, you will not be able to access the wealth of knowledge that is available. At every stage of your career, you need to get out of the trenches and talk to people who have done it before you. They can often give you well-grounded advice which you can accept or not, but at least you have heard it.

Mentorship for Focused Research Training

When you are thinking about going from your fellowship to do additional research training, your current mentors can give you ideas about which laboratories might be appropriate for you. They can make phone calls to the heads of these laboratories and put in a good word for you. Mentors who have developed a relationship with you over the years are more than happy to provide reference letters for you. These reference letters are crucial when you are looking for a research training position.

When you are looking for a mentor to be your laboratory supervisor, additional considerations come into play. For example, you are likely to spend a year or more with this individual. Do they have the characteristics which will allow you to establish a personal relationship with them? What is their relationship with other individuals in their laboratory? What is their relationship with other individuals in their institution? A formal supervisor, in addition to being a mentor, needs to have resources available for you. These resources include work facilities, funding for you to go to courses, conferences, and meetings, the ability to help you obtain salary support for your training as well as funding to do your research projects.

Typically, when you are ready to begin focused research training, there are several different laboratories in which you could work. You need to sit down with the directors of these laboratories and have frank discussions about your career aspirations. Over the course of these discussions, you can see if these individuals are empathetic, whether you think that they would be good mentors, and whether they have the time to spend with you. It is also important for you to speak with individual members of the various laboratories you are considering. They have already had extensive interactions with their laboratory directors, and they can tell you whether these individuals are good mentors or not. However, you should be aware that just because a mentor is good for one individual does not mean that they are good for another. You need to consider which of your needs they can address. If you ultimately find yourself in a situation where your mentor is not providing you with what you need, you should gracefully and diplomatically acquire a new mentor and sometimes even change laboratories.

Mentorship for New Physician-Scientists

As you become more senior, mentorship becomes more informal, and you need to proactively seek out mentors. When I came back to McGill after training in the United States for years, I was at a new hospital, and I did not know any potential mentors. This was problematic for me when I started applying for grants. I did not have any experience writing grants, and there was no one that I knew to turn to for advice. In retrospect, I should have been much more proactive in developing a mentor. There were many successful physician-scientists at my institution who could have provided some much-needed mentorship. All I needed to do was get out of my office and go talk to them. Thus, at your own institution, you need to talk with various individuals to see whether they would be willing to give you feedback on some of your papers and grant applications. Many individuals will not have the time or will not be interested; one or two will. Only by talking to various individuals you can identify who will be a good mentor for you.

Keep in mind that some mentors are good for some things and some are good for others. For example, at my institution, we have a very senior emeritus individual who is very knowledgeable about the political process at regional and national funding agencies. He has not been an active physician-scientist for many years, but he still has many contacts at the regional and national levels, and he is a very clear-thinking individual. If I ever have a political or strategic issue, he is the one I go to for advice. For other concerns, I have other individuals to whom I can turn. You should think very carefully about who you have access to and what type of mentorship you need. You likely will need different mentors for different aspects of your career.

It is very important for a new physician-scientist to develop at least one mentor who is a physician-scientist at their own institution. When you are first starting, it is very difficult to juggle your research career, your clinical career, and your family.

It is very helpful to see first-hand someone a few years ahead of you who is at mid-career and who has done this successfully. By observing this individual, you can get a clearer view of where your career may be going in 5 or 10 years. Once you have an idea of where you want your career to go, you will have a better idea of how to navigate the system.

The physician-scientist career is fraught with ups and downs. At multiple times during your career, you are going to experience serious frustrations. It is difficult to face these alone. Having a mentor who has gone through the system can help you get an idea of what the problem is and how to overcome it. A mentor can provide guidance on how to accept and respond to criticism. They can give you advice on how to deal with senior collaborators and co-investigators. They can give you advice on how to deal with clinical issues. If you do not have enough protected time for research and you want to negotiate more time, they can give you ideas of how to go about this. If you are having difficulty being funded, they can look at your grant applications and give you an idea of what you should be doing or what you are missing. If your manuscripts are not getting accepted for publication, they can give you helpful suggestions. At every stage of your career, it is important to have an experienced mentor to talk to. It can be difficult to be a physician-scientist in isolation. Mentorship is important at all stages of your career. Even the most senior physician-scientists still have mentors with whom they discuss various issues. Thus, I would highly encourage you to develop a strong network of mentors as you go through your career.

Being a Mentor

As you make the transition from research trainee to physician-scientist, you also need to make the transition from mentee to mentor. All physician-scientists need to be active mentors for medical students, residents, fellows, graduate students, and other clinicians. It is part of your responsibility as a physician-scientist to be a good mentor (Table 15.1). Being a good mentor does not mean that you need to mentor everyone who approaches you or that you are suited to mentor everyone. Just as certain patients gravitate to certain doctors, certain students gravitate towards certain mentors. You may be a good mentor for one individual but not another. If you are a clinical epidemiologist, you may not be a good mentor for a PhD basic scientist. If you are a basic science researcher, you may not be a good mentor for a surgical resident who wants to do clinical research. When a student approaches you, it is important to speak with them at length and clarify for both of you whether a mentorship role would be appropriate. As a physician-scientist, you have developed knowledge and skills which are important to transmit to the next generation. However, you cannot spend all of your time being a mentor. You need to be selective about which mentees you take on and which you send on to others.

Table 15.1 Responsibilities of a mentor

Provide opportunities for mentee to:
Be first author on publications
Be involved in different types of studies
Gain administrative, research, and writing skills
Participate in all aspects of research
Network
Review manuscripts for journals
Discuss career development, family, and other matters
Facilitate mentee:
In obtaining salary support
In making contacts at your institution
In making contacts at conferences and meetings
By offering constructive feedback on their work
By making personal contact with possible job contacts/supervisors
By providing reference letters

What Makes a Good Mentor?

We rarely get any formal training in how to be a good mentor. For most of us, it is a question of experience. We have developed relationships with many mentors over the course of our clinical and research training. We try to avoid the bad and emulate the good.

From our bad experiences, it is important to examine why our relationship was less than optimal. In my experience, the primary reason was that the mentor's heart was not in it. There are many individuals who look like good mentors on paper but who do not have good mentorship skills. They often have a limited amount of time to fulfill their current responsibilities, and they do not have the time or are unwilling to make the time to mentor others. They are busy with their own research projects, clinical activities, and family responsibilities.

Our experiences with good mentors give us much to emulate. Good mentors are willing to share their time. They are no less overwhelmed with research responsibilities, clinical activities, and family commitments, yet they are willing to take time away from their work to help develop the careers of younger individuals. They recognize that it is important to help the next generation of physician-scientists as the previous generation helped them. Good mentors may not have their doors open 24 hours a day, but they do provide regular access. When they are with you, they listen. They are not distracted by phone calls and other individuals coming in the door. They can have the occasional coffee and discuss peripheral issues not directly related to research. They are willing to give career advice. They are willing to share their experiences and themselves. They give the impression that they remember what it was like when they were sitting in the trainee's place. Good mentors are friendly, enthusiastic, intelligent, experienced, and willing to share their knowledge. They do not think of the mentorship role as a burden.

Benefits of Being a Mentor

It is very fulfilling to see your mentees develop into excellent physicians, excellent scientists, and independent investigators. As an example, I have had a long relationship with one of my graduate students. This individual came to me as an undergraduate, and he wanted to do research in my laboratory. He excelled, and I encouraged him to go on to graduate studies in epidemiology. He did his Masters of Science in Epidemiology and subsequently completed his PhD. He has now moved on to a post-doctoral position in another city. We have worked together for over seven years. Before going on to his post-doctoral training, he was the manager of my laboratory. I feel that I transferred much of my knowledge about writing and grantsmanship to him. When he reviews a paper by one of my younger trainees, his comments are very similar to mine. Even though he has now moved on, we still collaborate on many projects. He is just on the verge of becoming a principal investigator in his own right. I am very proud to see what he has accomplished, and I think that I have had a hand in his development. When I look at his papers, I see my influence, and it is very gratifying. I know that long after I retire, he will be a productive researcher and will go on to help train the next generation of physician-scientists.

Reflections on Mentorship

I am now at mid-career and have been a physician-scientist at McGill University for over 15 years. I have been a mentor for scores of individuals, including undergraduate students, medical students, residents, fellows, research trainees, graduate students, and other clinicians. Some have come to me for supervision of research projects, and others have come to me for mentorship not directly related to a research project. Occasionally, I have had a bad situation, but overall it has been extremely positive. When I look at the students who have come through my laboratory, I am very proud. I see individuals who I mentored before they began medical school and who are now in practice. Some of these individuals are performing research. Some have gone on to do graduate studies in epidemiology or in public health. Some have made important contributions to the literature. Two of my research assistants married each other and are now parents. I have been invited by my students to weddings and to parties celebrating births. I have developed close relationships with many of the individuals that I have helped to mentor. Besides being a responsibility, it has been a pleasure to help in the development of these students. I really enjoy seeing young people blossom and surpass me. It is important to me that I am helping to train the next generation of physician-scientists. Even if my trainees go on to become 100% clinicians and do not take part in any research whatsoever, I think that their clinical skills are enhanced by the experiences that they have had in my laboratory. If you have a narrow view and are focused only on your own research projects, I think you are missing the big picture. You can have a much greater impact on the health of your community and your nation by training individuals who will have an impact themselves. These trainees will go on to train other trainees. In this way, you can have a far-reaching influence, much beyond that of your own laboratory. For these reasons, I find it very gratifying to be a mentor. I do not begrudge the time. It is difficult to juggle mentoring along with research, clinical, and family responsibilities, but I think being a mentor is an extremely important responsibility.

Summary

The topic of mentorship is both important and complex. It is not an exact science. In this chapter, I have tried to give you some of my thoughts about it. It is important for you to cultivate good mentors as you go along your career path. Once you become a physician-scientist, you have a responsibility to mentor other individuals. You have developed a wealth of knowledge and skills over the course of your training, and it is important that you share this with developing physician-scientists. We have chosen to become physician-scientists because we want to improve patient care and the overall health of the community. We can do this much more effectively by mentoring individuals who will eventually surpass us. We can achieve much greater impact by passing on our knowledge and experience than we can by exclusively focusing on our own research agendas. I would highly encourage you to cultivate good mentors over the course of your own career and to take the knowledge gained from these interactions to become a good mentor in your own right. Most physician-scientists have little formal training in mentorship. By emulating your effective mentors and by avoiding the mistakes made by your poor mentors, you will become a good mentor for the next generation of physician-scientists.

Key Points

- Mentors are helpful at every stage of your career.
- You need different types of mentors at different stages of your career.
- A single mentor cannot provide you with all the knowledge and skills you need to succeed.
- Keep in contact with past mentors; they can be valuable resources.
- The interests of mentor and mentee need to be in sync.
- When you are a mentor, make sure your mentees are involved in multiple aspects of the research process.
- Having both clinical and research exposure is valuable for the mentee.
- Mentors need to be available to their mentees.
- When you become a mentor, emulate the good qualities of your own mentors.

Suggested Reading

1. Barishansky RM. Paying it forward. The importance of being a mentor. Emerg Med Serv 2006; 35: 79.
2. Barkun A. Maximizing the relationship with a mentor. Gastrointest Endosc 2006; 64: S4–S6.
3. Bettmann M. Choosing a research project and a research mentor. Circulation 2009; 119: 1832–1835.
4. Kjeldsen K. A proficient mentor is a must when starting up with research. Exp Clin Cardiol 2006; 11: 243–245.
5. Lee JM, Anzai Y, Langlotz CP. Mentoring the mentors: aligning mentor and mentee expectations. Acad Radiol 2006; 13: 556–561.
6. Marks MB, Goldstein R. The mentoring triad: mentee, mentor, and environment. J Rheumatol 2005; 32: 216–218.
7. Omary MB. Mentoring the mentor: another tool to enhance mentorship. Gastroenterology 2008; 135: 13–16.
8. Reckelhoff JF. How to choose a mentor. Physiologist 2008; 51: 152–154.
9. Stone C. The importance of having a mentor, and how to find one. Gastrointest Endosc 2006; 63: 112–113.
10. White SJ, Tryon JE. How to find and succeed as a mentor. Am J Health Syst Pharm 2007; 64: 1258–1259.

Chapter 16
Lectures and Presentations

*When I give a lecture, I accept that people look at their watches,
but what I do not tolerate is when they look at it and raise it to
their ear to find out if it has stopped.*

–Marcel Achard

Introduction

Giving lectures and presentations is an important part of your career as a physician-scientist. Unfortunately, most physician-scientists have no formal training in lecturing. You can improve your lecturing skills with practice. There are tips and techniques that will help you prepare and deliver professional presentations. These methods can be learned from courses and books that focus on how to lecture. I encourage you, early in your career, to attend a course and/or read a book on improving your lecturing skills. In addition, examine the techniques of others when you attend their lectures and presentations.

During your career, you will be called upon to lecture in different settings. These include academic seminars, divisional rounds, grand rounds, industry events, job talks, late-breaking clinical trial sessions, original research sessions at national and international meetings, research rounds, scientific and professional meetings, and presentations to non-physicians and non-scientists. Each setting requires different lecturing and presentation styles. In this chapter, I suggest general tips for preparing and delivering lectures and presentations. I also provide advice on oral abstract presentations and full-length lectures. These formats apply to most of the presentations you will deliver in your career, regardless of the setting. Finally, I offer suggestions on how to lead question-and-answer sessions following your presentations, as well as tips about ancillary issues.

General Tips

Though your preparation and style of delivery may vary for different types of presentations, the following tips will help improve the clarity and professionalism of your presentation, regardless of the format or context (Table 16.1). Virtually all

M.J. Eisenberg, *The Physician Scientist's Career Guide*,
DOI 10.1007/978-1-60327-908-6_16, © Springer Science+Business Media, LLC 2011

Table 16.1 Tips for effective lectures and presentations

---
1. Tailor the amount of material to your time slot
2. Arrive early
3. Ensure you know how to use the microphone, projector, remote control, etc.
4. Begin with an overview of what you plan to cover
5. Make eye contact with audience members
6. Speak loudly and clearly
7. Modulate your voice, move around, and use body language
8. Use humor or emotion to break monotony
9. Consider the level of knowledge of your audience
10. Use examples to situate your theory in concrete terms
11. Encourage participation through questions or discussions
12. Leave time for questions, comments, and clarifications

---

lectures you give during your career will involve the use of slides. In other areas, such as the humanities, lectures are often delivered without slides. However, this type of presentation is uncommon for the physician-scientist.

There are formatting requirements to keep in mind for your slides. For example, make sure that each slide has adequate margins. Occasionally, you will present in a room where the screen is smaller than expected. If you do not have a large enough margin around your slides, some of your text and/or images will be cut off. In addition, use a large font, or your slides will not be visible to much of your audience. This is true for text slides as well as table and figure slides. The color scheme of your slides and the layout of the text should make them as easy to read as possible. Each slide should contain a title that encapsulates the message of that slide. Appropriate references should appear in small font at the bottom of the slide.

The use of slides should complement and enhance your lecture rather than detract from it. There is nothing worse than attending a lecture where the lecturer has obviously not spent time preparing the slides. The lecturer overwhelms you with too many slides, with too much detail, and with slides that are incoherent and lack a logical flow. It is frustrating for the audience when you have to rush through your presentation or when you have too much material left near the end of the lecture and need to skip slides.

Be in control during your presentation. Your presentation should be rehearsed in advance so that it is well paced and provides plenty of time for questions and discussion. When you minimize and simplify your slides, you will be able to speak at a reasonable pace. The audience will be able to follow what you say and absorb the relevant information. Show your audience that you respect them by preparing your slides in advance and making them easy to understand (Fig. 16.1). In the following sections, I present detailed tips that will improve the overall coherence of your presentation.

Use Uniform Structure

For clarity and coherence, use a uniform structure when creating your slide presentation. Slides should use the same format: font size, background color, and margins.

a. Effective Lecture Slides   **b. Poor Lecture Slides**

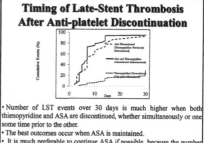

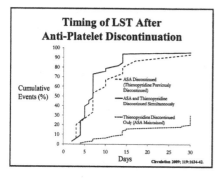

Fig. 16.1 Example Slides

The format of tables and figures should also be consistent. If you take slides from different lectures to create a new lecture, ensure that formatting is harmonious. The use of a uniform structure throughout your lecture demonstrates that you are a well-organized and logical individual. Even if your lecture itself is excellent, disjointed and disorganized slides detract from the audience's understanding. If abbreviations are used in one place but not in others, if margin sizes are different on some slides than others, if full sentences are used in some but not others, it will be apparent to an experienced observer and will detract from your presentation.

Minimize Your Slides

No matter what venue you are speaking in, limit the number of slides. A good rule of thumb is to use no more than one slide per minute. For example, in a one-hour time slot, you will often start 5 minutes late and need 10 minutes for questions. As a result, plan your presentation to be 45 minutes in length and use a maximum of 45 slides. Do not forget the time you allot for a question-and-answer period when deciding how many slides to create for your presentation. Using more than one slide per minute is a disservice to your audience. Although you are familiar with your material, the audience may not be. They cannot follow a large number of slides over a short period of time. Give them time to digest the contents of each slide and internalize what you are saying.

Although it may be difficult to limit yourself to one slide per minute, your audience will appreciate it. You will always have a lot more to say than there is time to present, but you need to prioritize and select only the most important information. Your audience will only take away a few points from your talk. As a result, there is no reason to overwhelm them with too many slides and details that will obscure the important points you want them to remember.

Simplify and Reduce the Number of Text Slides

In addition to limiting the number of slides you use, increase the clarity of your presentation by limiting the number of text slides. Text slides are the least effective method of getting your information to the audience. A successful presentation includes tables and figures. You can also include pictures. Present an eclectic collection of slides to maintain the audience's interest and facilitate their understanding.

When you do include text slides, keep the number of words on each slide to a minimum. Reading your slides to the audience is dull and ineffective. Slides should jog your memory and help the audience focus on important points. They should not contain paragraphs or full sentences that you repeat to the audience. Include no more than four or five lines per slide and do not use full sentences. Instead, use a bullet format with words or phrases. These should be reminders of the points you want to make. The majority of the information you convey should not come from text slides; rather, it should come from you and from tables and figures.

Use Tables and Figures to Illustrate Important Information

Using tables and figures breaks up a monotonous presentation, making the lecture more visually interesting and more likely to retain the attention of the audience. Tables and figures illustrate the content of your presentation in a precise manner that will be easier for your audience to follow.

Tables are an effective medium for concisely communicating results to an audience. A simple table helps audiences quickly understand the point you are making. A common mistake is to present too much information in tables; when this occurs, the audience cannot absorb the content. Keep the number of columns and rows to a minimum; no more than four or five columns and four or five rows. The information on each slide should be kept to a minimum, and the audience should be allowed at least 1 minute to view the slide and internalize the information. You should never say, "I know you can't read all the information on this slide but. . . ." Instead, reduce the information on each slide to the essential points you want to convey. If you are not going to mention it during your talk, there is no reason to present it on the slide.

Summarize the information in the table rather than reading out every number; the audience can read it for themselves. Instead, be analytical. Rather than saying that the average age of females was 75 and the average age of males was 72, you can say that, on average, females were three years older than males. Do not present a text slide after each table or figure to summarize the previous slide. It is much more effective to verbalize the results while you are presenting the table or figure. This allows the audience to visualize what you are saying.

You can reduce the amount of information on each slide in a number of other ways. For example, if all the numbers in your table are percentage points, do not put a percent sign after each number. Instead, put the percent sign in parentheses at the top of the column. Use abbreviations when your audience is knowledgeable in the area you are presenting. However, do not use abbreviations when some of your audiences are not familiar with your terminology. It is frustrating to attend a lecture where the lecturer uses abbreviations that you are not familiar with.

Figures are also very effective for conveying information. Use one figure per slide, and maximize the size of the figure so that it is clearly visible. Figures should be simple. Walk your audience through the figures as you give the lecture. Mention what the slide is about and define the X- and Y-axes for graphs and the columns and rows for tables before presenting the data itself. When preparing a figure, ensure that labels for the X- and Y-axes are easily legible. Be careful when using figures directly from journal articles. The legend for the Y-axis is usually small, vertical, and illegible. The legend for Y-axes should be presented horizontally so that it is easily readable by the audience, including those at the back of the room. Color can increase the clarity of figures and help maintain audience interest. Remember to keep it simple!

Lecturing

Most physician-scientists get insufficient experience lecturing during their training. However, you will be required to give many lectures during your career. As you become increasingly senior, your audience will increase in size. At the beginning of your career, spend time rehearsing your lectures in advance. This will be helpful once you become more senior. It is often helpful to present lectures to your research group before presenting them in public. Rehearsing helps iron out problems that you were not aware of and helps identify inconsistencies. It also helps with timing and pacing. Obtain feedback from your research team to improve your lecture before presenting to a more critical audience. Although it is natural to be nervous when you first start lecturing, you will become more and more at ease as you advance in your career. The best method for reducing your anxiety is to rehearse your presentation.

Oral Abstracts

You will present many oral abstracts during your career. Oral abstracts are the typical format for presenting research findings at national and international conferences.

Similar to abstracts of published articles, an oral abstract provides a brief overview of the background of and rationale for addressing your research question and identifies your objectives, methods, results, and conclusions. As you become more senior, many of your students and trainees will present oral abstracts. As a result, you should become an expert in this type of presentation. Generally, you have a 10–15 minutes time slot for an oral abstract. If you have 15 minutes, this usually includes 12 minutes of presentation followed by a 3-minutes question-and-answer period. Therefore, you should have no more than 12 slides.

I always use the same format when preparing slides for an oral abstract presentation. The first slide is the Title slide. The title should be large and succinct. The middle of the slide has your name and degrees. The bottom of the slide has the location of your institution and coordinates. At the very bottom of the slide is your disclosure statement. This reminds you to present any potential conflicts of interest you might have. The second and third slides present the Background section. These slides are usually text slides. Next, depending on the presentation, you will need two or three Methods slides. These are typically presented in text format as well. For an oral abstract presentation of 12 minutes, presenting more than three Methods slides will prevent you from spending adequate time on your results. In the Methods section, use subtitles such as Patient Population, Intervention, and Statistical Analysis to orient the audience.

The bulk of the presentation should focus on your results. Typically, include four or five slides in this section. Results slides should be presented in a format that is parallel to the Methods section. That is, the first Results slide should deal with the first subtitle that was presented in the first Methods slide. If the subtitle in that section was "Patient Population," the first Results slide should be the same and so on. If you need to present a lot of information about patient population, you may require two slides. The title of the second slide could read "Patient Population (Continued)." The bulk of your Results slides should deal with the analyses involved. They should be presented in a logical manner.

The first Analysis slide should be a general descriptive analysis. It should be followed by more specific analyses. If it is a basic science presentation, results of each experiment should be presented in chronological order or in the order that makes the most logical sense. Each Results slide should deal with one topic. Since these slides are the most complex, you may want to spend more than 1 minute on each slide with slightly less than 1 minute on earlier Background and Methods slides. It is important that you do not rush through the Results slides. Whenever possible, results should be presented in tables or figures, since they will be more easily understood by the audience. Following the Results slides, if time permits, include a Limitations slide. This information should be presented on one slide. After presenting each potential limitation, discuss how you dealt with it in the analysis or why you believe it did not impact on the conclusions.

The final slide(s) are the Discussion or Conclusion slides. They are usually presented in text format. Emphasize the major conclusions at this point. Each slide should deal with your take-home message and big picture. Details should have been presented in the Results section. Therefore, if there are any trends you want your audience to understand or associations you want them to know, present these during the Results slides. Conclusions slides should deal with the big picture. Does the information reflect previous or current research? How should this information affect clinical practice? What are future areas of research that need to be further explored?

At the end, include a slide listing co-investigators, research assistants, and laboratory technicians who contributed to the study. Following the presentation, have several blank slides ready. When the presentation is finished and you have thanked the audience, project a blank slide. It is distracting to the audience to have a projection of your Conclusions slide during the discussion period. Following two or three blank slides, keep your backup slides. These should include important information that you might be questioned about. Include no more than two or three backup slides so that you do not have search through all your extra slides to find the one you are looking for.

Be an expert at preparing slides for oral abstract presentations and at presenting in this format. Be precise, succinct, clear, and coherent in your message. This applies to both your oral presentation and your slides. The ability to present clearly is a neglected area in research training, and I encourage you to become expert at it early in your career.

Full-Length Lectures

Full-length lectures should use the techniques previously discussed. Most full-length lectures are allotted a 1-h time slot. Lectures often begin 5 or 10 minutes late, and you need to leave 5 or 10 minutes at the end for questions. Consequently, present no more than 45 slides in a one-hour time slot so that you do not have to rush the audience through the material. The nature of your presentation needs to be adapted to the audience. If this is a research presentation, it should follow the above-mentioned oral abstract presentation format. While most of your presentation should focus on your own research, you need to present it in the context of previous research in the area.

Following the Title slide, an extensive Background section should detail information that puts your research in context. Therefore, prepare 10–15 slides of background information for a 45-min talk. Ideally, these should consist of tables and figures from previous studies. Background slides need to be presented in a coherent and logical order. Following the Background section, present a list of your objectives and hypotheses in bullet format. Just like an original research article, the structure of a full-length research presentation should be like an hourglass. The beginning of the talk should be broad and general, and your research question should represent the narrow part of the hourglass.

The Methods and Results sections should be adjusted to the type of information you are presenting. If the focus of the presentation is one single study, the format used for oral abstract presentations can be used. For other types of presentations, present your audience with a series of experiments or related studies. In this case, the most coherent way to organize the information is to have one or two Methods slides followed by slides of the Results of the study. Then you present the next study, and so on. It is not useful to detail the methods used for multiple experiments followed by the results of all experiments. This is confusing to the audience, and it may be unclear which methods and results were related.

In a 45-min presentation, devote 10–15 minutes to the Background section, 15–20 minutes to the Methods and Results sections, and 10–15 minutes to the Limitations, Discussion, and Conclusions sections. Your research should be put into context, both at the beginning and at the end of your presentation. Most of your audience will not be experts in your field. Ensure that they understand the rationale for the questions asked and the methods used. They need to see your research in the context of previous research and understand the significance of your research as it relates to current practice. You can also mention the next steps that need to be taken.

Question-and-Answer Session

At the end of most presentations, there is a question-and-answer session. Keep your answers brief and focused. This is an opportunity for the audience to express issues they need clarified; it is not the time to restate the conclusions of your study. Do not use the session as an opportunity to expound upon your subject matter. Use occasional backup slides but keep them to a minimum. Repeat questions that you do not think are audible to the audience, and ask for clarification when a question is unclear. It is helpful to paraphrase the question for the audience. If you do not know the answer to the question, be honest. State that you do not know the answer but that it is an interesting question that deserves future study. Do not be afraid to tell an audience member that they have posed an excellent question; they love to hear that. The bottom line is that you want the question-and-answer session to clarify your message, so ensure that speakers are heard, that the audience understands the questions, and that your answers provide new information on these points.

Ancillary Issues

An experienced lecturer is prepared for all eventualities. Therefore, arrive early to make sure that your equipment is in place and functioning. There is nothing more annoying to an audience than when a lecturer appears at the last minute only to find that the technical equipment is not ready. Arrive 10–15 minutes early and make sure that the equipment is set up and working properly.

Prepare the hardware and software you need ahead of time, and ensure that it works. Bring your own laser pointer, but minimize its use during your presentation. It is distracting for an audience when the lecturer is waving a laser pointer all over their slides during a presentation. Use the pointer briefly to highlight major points. Another useful piece of equipment to bring is a remote control for the laptop. These are inexpensive and often integrated with a laser pointer. Using a remote control gives you freedom of movement; you are not tethered to the computer. As a result, you can walk around during the presentation, which can be an effective means of gaining the audience's attention. Even when the sponsor provides a laptop and data projector, bring a backup laptop and a memory stick containing your presentation. Technical difficulties are common, and you need to be prepared for them. In addition, make sure to check the compatibility of any software you are using ahead of time. For example, make sure you have the correct version of Word, PowerPoint, or any other programs you are using. A computer that does not have the version of a program in which you created a document may not be able to open your document. Be aware that, if you created your PowerPoint presentation in one version, formatting may be altered and some features may not work another version. Finally, concentrate on keeping the audience engaged, and facilitate their understanding of your presentation.

Here are some tips and techniques to improve the clarity and interest of your presentation style.

- Always face your audience when speaking.
- Make sure that the computer screen is situated in such a way that you do not have to turn away from the audience to see your slides. Do not face the screen while talking.
- Do not speak in a monotone during the presentation; change the cadence of your speech occasionally.
- Speak clearly at a moderate pace.
- Use some hand motions.
- Make eye contact with the audience.
- Be animated, enthusiastic, and interested in your information.
- Ask the audience questions in a non-confrontational manner to engage their interest.
- Make sure your questions are simple and easily answered.
- If a member of the audience is an expert in the subject area, ask them a question during the course of the lecture.

Experiment with these techniques to engage your audience. You want to come across as an engaging, interesting, entertaining, and educational speaker so that you can share your passion for your research with the audience.

Summary

Giving lectures and presentations is an essential part of your career as a physician-scientist. It is not enough to perform research projects and publish results. You need to be active in translating that knowledge to clinicians who can make use of it. Many techniques can be used to improve your presentations and to make them more effective vehicles for transmitting information. When you pay attention to simple details, your lectures and presentations can be maximally effective. Although most physician-scientists do not receive formal training in lecturing skills, it is very worthwhile to acquire these skills. Not only do you want to be perceived as an excellent physician and scientist, you also want to be considered an excellent teacher and lecturer.

Key Points

- Take a course or read a book on how to improve your lecturing skills.
- Include a title and relevant citations on each slide.
- Employ uniform structure and formatting for your slides.
- Minimize the number of slides to one per minute.
- Slides should jog your memory, not list everything you want to say.
- Reduce the amount of information included in tables and figures to points you will actually discuss.
- Minimize abbreviations and jargon.
- Create your presentation in an "hourglass" format.
- Prepare for technical difficulties; bring a backup laptop and memory stick.
- Engage your audience by speaking clearly and animatedly.

Suggested Reading

1. Azer SA. What makes a great lecture? Use of lectures in a hybrid PBL curriculum. Kaohsiung J Med Sci 2009; 25: 109–115.
2. Balistreri WF. Giving an effective presentation. J Pediatr Gastroenterol Nutr 2002; 35: 1–4.
3. Bulska E. Good oral presentation of scientific work. Anal Bioanal Chem 2006; 385: 403–405.
4. Copeland HL, Longworth DL, Hewson MG, Stoller JK. Successful lecturing: a prospective study to validate attributes of the effective medical lecture. J Gen Intern Med 2000; 15: 366–371.
5. Gelula MH. Effective lecture presentation skills. Surg Neurol 1997; 47: 201–204.
6. Gelula MH. Preparing and organizing for a lecture. Surg Neurol 1997; 47: 86–88.
7. Hornick L. The lecturer and the lecture. J Med Educ 1986; 61: 858–859.
8. Jenkins JL Jr. In the spotlight. How to develop an effective public presentation. EMS Mag 2007; 36: 42–44.
9. Mann D. Guidelines for creating effective slides and overhead transparencies used for teaching. J Am Osteopath Assoc 1992; 92: 1526–1528.
10. Richardson D. Don't dump the didactic lecture; fix it. Adv Physiol Educ 2008; 32: 23–24.
11. Strasburger VC. Have jumpdrive, will travel: medical lecturing in the age of PowerPoint. Clin Pediatr (Phila) 2009; 48: 799–800.
12. Walker JD, Cotner SH, Baepler PM, Decker MD. A delicate balance: integrating active learning into a large lecture course. CBE Life Sci Educ 2008; 7: 361–367.

Chapter 17
Relations with Industry

Moderation in all things.
–Terence

Introduction

Relationships with the pharmaceutical and medical device industry are pervasive in the world of physician-scientists. These relationships can affect your research and promotions, in addition to posing a variety of ethical concerns. A full discussion of research ethics is beyond the scope of this book, but I suggest consulting the research ethics board at your institution to inform yourself of the regulations governing research ethics in general and relationships with industry in particular. Nevertheless, relationships with industry can be beneficial to your research program and can have a significant positive impact on public health. You need to have a solid understanding of the pros and cons of different types of industry relationships so that you can make informed decisions about when to become involved.

Types of Relationships

At its simplest, a relationship with the pharmaceutical or medical device industry might involve a company representative visiting you to discuss their products. Relationships can also include direct involvement in your work in the context of grant support, multi-center trials, or contract research. Speaker's bureaus and sponsored conferences or presentations might be less directly related to your research but might include a financial relationship with industry as well as a potential influence on your work.

Company Representatives

As a physician-scientist, you will often be in contact with representatives from pharmaceutical and medical device industries. At most hospitals, industry representatives are allowed to visit physicians to inform them about new developments.

M.J. Eisenberg, *The Physician Scientist's Career Guide,*
DOI 10.1007/978-1-60327-908-6_17, © Springer Science+Business Media, LLC 2011

In these situations, each physician has to decide whether to have direct contact with industry representatives. Representatives typically visit your office for short periods of time and present you with the latest data regarding their drug or device. However, meeting with a "rep" takes up time in your busy schedule. In addition, reps are not impartial about their product. Nevertheless, they can be helpful in some cases. For instance, they sometimes give you articles or refer you to data about the most recent research regarding their drug or device.

Some hospitals have policies prohibiting representatives from meeting with physicians. This type of policy has positive and negative aspects. The positive aspects are that conference agendas are not influenced by the company representative who is providing the accompanying meal. When representatives provide meals for conferences, the topic of the conferences is often influenced by which company is sponsoring the event. On the other hand, when no meal is provided, attendance is often sparse and the audience may be less attentive. Many physicians believe that they are not influenced by these types of interactions. However, research suggests that physicians are influenced by these events more than they realize.

Industry-Sponsored Presentations

As a physician-scientist, contact with industry representatives may have significant impacts beyond your research program and prescriptive practices. Since you are a qualified researcher, they may invite you to speak at local conferences. These talks usually address a particular drug or device the company produces or general information about the area in which their product is used.

Companies often sponsor a presentation at a nice local restaurant and invite clinicians to attend your presentation. They also provide you with an honorarium to defray the cost of your preparation and attendance. Representatives typically want your presentation to support the interests of their company. In my experience, they usually do not have a problem with your discussion of the limitations of their drug or device; they just want you to raise awareness of their product. However, even though they will not dictate what you say, you might have a subconscious or even conscious desire for the company representatives to approve of your presentation.

These types of conferences are popular among physician-scientists. For most of us, it is hard to turn down an honorarium and a quality meal. In addition, presenting a lecture is good for your CV. However, be aware of the ethical issues involved. For example, your presentation may influence other physicians to use a product or device. As a result, being biased because of a desire to please the representative might be a significant concern. Similarly, if you have a financial interest in the product, clearly disclose it so that your audience knows what perspective the information is coming from.

Speaker's Bureau

Pharmaceutical and medical device companies often keep lists of potential speakers. These are called speaker's bureaus. If you are a member of a speaker's bureau, the company will arrange for you to give presentations at hospitals around the country and sometimes overseas. These presentations are used to promote their drug or device. The more prominent you are, the more likely it is that you will be asked to be a member of a speaker's bureau. Giving presentations for drug and device companies can be remunerative. In addition, speaking at different institutions may look impressive on your CV. It helps demonstrate your national and international recognition. Nevertheless, there are ethical issues involved. The companies are not typically interested in flying you around to speak at different institutions unless you speak in favor of their product; so, be very objective in your presentation. If you cannot be objective, do not participate. You also need to consider that time spent on these activities takes time away from your peer-reviewed research activities. Therefore, although you may choose to do this on occasion, ensure that it is a minimal time commitment.

Investigator-Initiated Grants

Pharmaceutical and device companies sometimes provide limited grant support to physician-scientists. These grants are called "investigator-initiated" grants. The amount of funding available is often less than what you can obtain from a peer-reviewed funding agency. However, it is possible to obtain funding for a topic that might not be funded by a peer-reviewed agency. For example, peer-reviewed funding agencies often do not provide financial support to study a particular drug or device. If you are interested in studying that drug or device, the only way you may be able to obtain funding is from the company itself. In addition, grant support may sometimes be obtained faster from a pharmaceutical or device company than from a peer-reviewed funding agency. Be aware, however, that overhead costs and Institutional Review Board fees will be deducted from the budget you receive; account for this in your budget request.

Although industry funds may be useful and more rapidly obtainable, be aware that funding from a pharmaceutical or medical device company is not beneficial when it comes to promotion. Most career award committees at peer-reviewed funding agencies and most promotion committees at universities do not consider pharmaceutical or device company funding during their deliberations. In addition, the integrity of the work sponsored by industry may be called into question because of the influence a company might have on the objectivity of your research. As a result, although you might spend part of your time working on projects funded by industry, do not spend the bulk of your time on these activities. Certainly, at the beginning of your career, I would consider minimizing the amount of time you spend on industry-sponsored activities.

Of note, some peer-reviewed funding agencies will provide complementary support for an industry-funded project. Once your proposal is approved and you have obtained a written commitment for funding from a company, submit your proposal to the peer-reviewed funding agency. They may contribute additional funds for the project. The proposal goes through a regular peer-reviewed funding committee. If they approve funding, you will receive academic credit for your research.

In addition, consider applying to a peer-reviewed funding agency with an add-on study related to your industry-sponsored project. For example, if you have industry funding for a multi-center trial or cohort study, you may be able to obtain a peer-reviewed grant to collect blood on these patients to examine an additional topic of scientific interest. Complementary funding from a peer-reviewed funding agency will substantially improve your likelihood of a promotion, whereas a purely industry-sponsored study will not.

Multi-Center Trials

Pharmaceutical and medical device companies often sponsor large multi-center clinical trials. Involvement in these trials can be beneficial to your career when you are involved at the steering committee level. The publications that result from these trials often affect clinical practice and are published in high-impact journals. However, contributing patients to multi-center trials without being a co-author of any related publications is of limited value to your career. In addition, these trials require much of your time that could otherwise be spent on your own projects. Therefore, I would not spend an inordinate amount of your time during the early stages of your career on large multi-center trials unless you are on a steering committee. Even later on in your career, it is usually more beneficial to spend time on your own research, unless you really need the funding to maintain your research program. Reimbursement for enrolling patients in industry-sponsored trials can be substantial. However, reimbursement cannot be used to supplement your salary. These monies can be used only for research expenses (e.g., hiring research assistants and nurses, buying computers, attending meetings, etc.). If there is a dry period when you do not have much peer-reviewed funding, you could supplement your research budget program by enrolling patients in industry-sponsored trials. However, focus on your own research once you obtain adequate funding.

Contract Research and Consulting

Pharmaceutical and medical device companies sometimes offer opportunities for contract research and consulting. In these situations, they approach investigators to work on some aspect of the research agenda of the company. These relationships are remunerative but are not typically useful for advancing your career. If the projects have intellectual content that is scientifically sound, it might be worthwhile to have part of your research program funded as contract research. However, if the bulk of your research is contract research, it is unlikely that your applications for career awards or promotions will be successful.

If you choose to do contract research with a particular company, make it clear in the contract that you retain the ability to publish the results regardless of the outcome. In addition, as part of your contract, obtain a commitment that you can use the acquired data for additional projects. For example, if you assemble a large registry for a company to examine a particular issue, you may be able to use the same database to study other issues once your report is completed. This strategy could prove fruitful, particularly when the project would not be funded by a peer-reviewed funding agency. To ensure that the contract is sound and allows you the freedom to perform high-quality research, have one of your mentors and one of your institution's lawyers examine the contract before signing it.

Sponsorship for Conferences, Workshops, and Seminars

Pharmaceutical and medical device companies often reserve a certain percentage of their budget to promote educational activities for physicians. If you approach them at the right time in their budget cycle, they may have funds available to sponsor conferences, workshops, and seminars. If there is a particular conference or seminar, you would like to host, approach them and request funding. There are obvious ethical issues regarding receiving such support. Make it clear that the intellectual content of your conference will be independent of their funding. This is called an "unrestricted educational grant". The company gives you the money, and you control the content of the conference, workshop, or seminar. These funds can help you organize a conference that otherwise would not be feasible.

Conflicts of Interest

When you accept funding from a pharmaceutical or medical device company, it might be perceived as a potential conflict of interest with respect to publishing articles on related topics. Virtually all journals require that you report any potential conflict of interest (Table 17.1) when you submit a manuscript. This includes relevant interactions that are not directly related to your work but that might influence your interpretation of the data. Most journals require you to report any relationship that may influence the way your work is presented to an audience, regardless of whether these relationships have ended by the time you submit the manuscript.

Many journals require that you identify any relationships or interests that took place over the three–five years prior to submission, and will also instruct you to disclose interactions that occurred outside that time frame when they might have influenced your work. This is a laudatory practice. Nevertheless, simply reporting a potential conflict of interest may not be enough. Since you have a financial relationship with the company, you might not be completely impartial in reporting the advantages and limitations of their drug or device. As a result, I would try to avoid writing about topics for which you have a conflict of interest. If you own stock in or have a financial relationship with a particular company, avoid developing that area as part of your research.

Table 17.1 Potential conflicts of interest with industry & disclosure procedures

Potential conflicts of interest	Where and how to disclose conflicts of interest
Awards Co-development of a product Consulting fees Employment Expert testimony Financial or other relationship with your spouse or children Honoraria Membership in an advocacy group Other financial relationships Patents or royalties related to area of study Payment for writing a manuscript Personal relationships Research program initiated by a company Speaker's bureaus Sponsorship for meetings/lectures Stocks Support for travel Support for research	• Abstracts: – Written disclosure when submitting to meetings or journals • Articles: – Written disclosure when submitting for publication – Usually on the title page or in acknowledgements – Be specific about the role of a funding organization or sponsor • Poster: – Written disclosure on poster • Presentations: – Written disclosure on first slide – Mention during presentation • Disclose any relationship, even when it is not considered a conflict of interest • If you have nothing to disclose, state this

1. Journal of the American Medical Association. JAMA Instructions for Authors. http://jama.ama-assn.org/misc/ifora.dtl#ConflictsofInterestandFinancialDisclosures. Accessed March 10, 2010.
2. New England Journal of Medicine. Author Center Help. http://authors.nejm.org/Help/acHelp.asp. Accessed March 10, 2010.

Another area where physician-scientists sometimes have relationships with industry is the co-development of a new drug or device. Some physician-scientists develop products in conjunction with a company. The physician-scientist receives financial support from the company for their research and has an equity interest in the company. As long as your relationships with the company are completely transparent, this is an acceptable practice. When developing a new drug or device, physician-scientists often have difficulty obtaining funding from peer-reviewed funding agencies; as a result, working with a company can be beneficial. However, make it clear to those involved that there is a financial relationship between you and the company. In addition, be aware that this type of activity may not be as highly valued by career award and promotion committees as peer-reviewed research.

Ethics

Ethical issues need to be addressed when dealing with pharmaceutical and medical device companies. A full discussion of these issues is beyond the scope of this book. Nevertheless, I would advise you to proceed with caution in your relationships with industry. At the beginning of your career, try to minimize your relationships with industry until you have a good grasp of the ethical issues. If you have concerns, consult your ethics review board and your mentors before committing yourself. There are positive and negative aspects of relationships with industry. You do not want to develop a relationship that you will later regret. All universities have regulations governing relationships with industry. These regulations govern patents, accepting funding from industry, and how much time you can spend as a consultant. Review them before getting involved.

Summary

A certain amount of interaction with industry can be beneficial, although many of the activities you can engage in with pharmaceutical and device companies are not useful for promotional purposes or for obtaining career awards. However, industry contracts can occasionally complement your peer-reviewed funding. In some cases, industry support can allow you to do research that you would not be able to perform otherwise. Before you embark on a relationship with industry, obtain the opinions of your senior colleagues and consult your institution's regulations.

Key Points

- Be aware of potential conflicts of interest and ethical issues in your relations with industry.
- Review regulations of your institution regarding involvement with industry.
- Relationships can include interactions with pharmaceutical and medical device representatives, involvement in industry-sponsored presentations, conferences, seminars, speaker's bureaus, multi-center trials, contract research, consulting, or investigator-initiated grants.
- Relationships with industry can compromise your objectivity.
- Consider investigator-initiated grants for projects that will not be funded by peer-reviewed funding organizations.
- Consider the time required before committing.
- Do not spend time on industry commitments at the expense of your other work.
- Limit your involvement to that which is beneficial to your research and career.
- Disclose any relationships that may have a bearing on your work in all publications and presentations.

Suggested Readings

1. Bhandari M, Busse JW, Jackowski D, et al. Association between industry funding and statistically significant pro-industry findings in medical and surgical randomized trials. CMAJ 2004;170: 477–480.
2. Bhandari M, Jonsson A, Buhren V. Conducting industry-partnered trials in orthopaedic surgery. Injury 2006; 37: 361–366.

3. Fox JE. Investigative partnership with industry. Invest Radiol 1993; 28 (Suppl 2): S41–S43.
4. Gozzani JL. Ethics Committee, conflict of interest, and registry of clinical assays. Rev Bras Anestesiol 2008; 58: 91–94.
5. Jorgensen AW, Maric KL, Tendal B, Faurschou A, Gotzsche PC. Industry-supported meta-analyses compared with meta-analyses with non-profit or no support: differences in methodological quality and conclusions. BMC Med Res Methodol 2008; 8: 60.
6. Psaty BM. Conflict of interest, disclosure, and trial reports. JAMA 2009; 301: 1477–1479.
7. Rasmussen N. The drug industry and clinical research in interwar America: three types of physician collaborator. Bull Hist Med 2005; 79: 50–80.
8. Rothman DJ, McDonald WJ, Berkowitz CD, et al. Professional medical associations and their relationships with industry: a proposal for controlling conflict of interest. JAMA 2009; 301: 1367–1372.
9. Saidman LJ. Unresolved issues relating to peer review, industry support of research, and conflict of interest. Anesthesiology 1994; 80: 491–492.
10. Tereskerz PM, Hamric AB, Guterbock TM, Moreno JD. Prevalence of industry support and its relationship to research integrity. Account Res 2009; 16: 78–105.

Part IV
Parting Words of Advice – Putting It All Together

Life is like riding a bicycle. To keep your balance, you must keep moving.

–Albert Einstein

Chapter 18
Balancing Research, Clinical Activities, and Family Life

> *Organization is not an option, it is a fundamental survival skill and distinct competitive advantage.*
> –Pam N. Woods

Introduction

Balancing your research activities, clinical activities, and family life can be one of the most challenging aspects of being a physician-scientist. Both your career and your family require substantial time commitments. Besides being a good scientist and a good physician, you want to be a good spouse and a good parent. If you devote all your time to being a good physician-scientist, your family life will suffer. If you devote all your time to your family life, your career will flounder. Achieving the right balance is a difficult task. Time management and the ability to delegate effectively are important skills to develop in order to balance these important areas. In this chapter, I discuss some of the issues you may face and provide strategies that I have found useful. I recognize that there is great variety in people's family structures, but my experience in balancing a physician-scientist career with other aspects of my life has largely revolved around my wife and children, so my discussion reflects this. In addition, many of the tips I suggest for organizing and prioritizing your activities are applicable to any activities you might want to fit into your schedule, whether a spouse and children are part of the equation or not. I recommend that you read one of the many comprehensive books on time management in addition to this chapter; different techniques work for different people, but everyone needs to identify strategies that work best for them.

Balancing Work and Family Activities

It is important to establish your research program and productivity early in your career. These activities require that you spend long hours doing research. However, you also need to make sure that you have adequate time to spend with your family.

M.J. Eisenberg, *The Physician Scientist's Career Guide*,
DOI 10.1007/978-1-60327-908-6_18, © Springer Science+Business Media, LLC 2011

At the beginning of your career, you may find yourself spending long hours at the hospital and at your laboratory, leaving early in the morning and arriving home late at night. If this situation develops, you will have minimal interaction with your spouse and your children. You may end up not doing many of the chores at home, and you will not be viewed as an active member of your family. If you arrive home late every night, you will be unable to eat dinner with your family, help with homework, or play ball with your children. As much as possible, try to return home in time to have dinner with your family, participate in evening activities with your children, and spend quality time with your partner. You can work later that night when your children are in bed or set aside time on the weekends.

Several strategies can help you maximize the quality time you spend with your family. First, develop "protected time" for your partner and children. My wife and I try to go out every Thursday night. That is our regular date night. It is important to spend time alone with your spouse. It is easy to get so busy with professional and child-related activities that you lose touch with your spouse. Make sure this does not happen. Similarly, it is important to set aside time for family activities on weekends. This can be difficult if you and your partner are frequently on call. Either my wife or I, and sometimes both of us, are often on call. Nevertheless, we find time to do family activities together. This may involve cross-country skiing on a Sunday afternoon, going on a hike, going to a museum, or going out to dinner. Whatever the activity is, it is very important that you spend quality time together as a family on a regular basis. Plan ahead, and take advantage of time when everyone is available.

Second, you must be willing to delegate many childcare and household activities (Table 18.1). Cooking, cleaning, and laundry are all activities that need to be performed on a regular basis in every household. However, these activities do not constitute quality time with your spouse and children. If you and your spouse have full-time careers, you will benefit from employing someone to do at least some of these chores for you. If you have a young family, I highly encourage you to get a

Table 18.1 Tasks you can delegate

At work	At home
1. Assigning tasks to team members	1. Basic childcare
2. Checking guidelines for journals, funding agencies, etc.	2. Cleaning
3. Creating PowerPoint presentations	3. Food preparation
4. Doing literature searches	4. Grocery shopping
5. Filing	5. Laundry
6. Preparing first drafts of letters and grants	6. Repairs
7. Investigating funding opportunities	7. Running errands
8. Making travel arrangements	8. Yard work
9. Opening and sorting mail	9. Taxes
10. Ordering supplies	
11. Ordering/retrieving articles	
12. Sending mail, faxes, etc.	
13. Proof-reading and formatting documents	

full-time nanny; it certainly helped us a lot. The nanny can do the cooking, cleaning, laundry, and grocery shopping. If you have young children at home, the nanny can look after them in a professional manner. If your children are in daycare, she can pick them up and bring them home. When at work, you can concentrate on your research and clinical activities, knowing with confidence that your children are well cared for and that household activities are under control. Full-time nannies can be expensive, but your income as a physician-scientist is more than sufficient to absorb the cost. Certainly, in the early years of your family, this expense is justified. As your children grow older and do not require such close supervision, you may be able to make do with part-time help. Nevertheless, if both you and your spouse are working, professional help at home will help you maximize your quality time with your family. In addition to hiring a nanny, you can employ others to take care of your garden, remove the snow, clean the house, do your taxes, or any of the other tasks that eat into your time with your family.

A third strategy is to make sure that you and your spouse are equally involved in household activities. This may include doing homework with the children, cleaning up on weekends, going shopping, etc. Every couple has a different breakdown in terms of who does what. Have a frank discussion with your spouse about what each person's responsibilities are. Someone needs to be responsible for childcare arrangements, and someone needs to be responsible for household repairs. Who is responsible for bill payments, taxes, investments, going to parent–teacher meetings, and buying clothes for the children? These issues and many more need to be discussed so that one individual does not end up taking on the majority of the household responsibilities. Your spouse needs to be engaged in this process. When your children are old enough, they can perform their share of the household duties as well. Older children can keep their rooms clean, prepare their own breakfasts, and look after their younger siblings. This is helpful to you and an effective way to maximize the time your family has to spend together once chores are done. It also gives children a sense of responsibility and maturity.

Fourth, you also need to be creative about resolving scheduling issues. There are occasions when my wife is rounding at the hospital and I am on call for interventional cardiology. When I am called, I have to be in the hospital within 20 minutes. In the past, I was sometimes faced with the situation where I had five children and no babysitter or no way to get them to school. You need to anticipate these problems and have contingency plans in place. Perhaps your children can take the bus, walk to school, or ride their bikes instead. Thankfully, our oldest daughter is now old enough to babysit!

Finally, as much as possible, delegate nonessential activities at work to reserve as much time as possible for "creative" activities, including paper writing, grant writing, and developing new research ideas (Table 18.1). For instance, to see whether an idea you are considering for a meta-analysis is feasible, a research assistant could do the preliminary literature search. Your research assistants can also write drafts of letters, grant proposals, and budgets. They can research funding opportunities or proofread manuscripts. This will free up of time during which you can focus on things that require your personal attention. Carefully consider what can be delegated, and be as organized as possible to make sure that you have free time to spend with your family.

Starting a Family

Your family is a critical part of your life. For most of us, our families are more important than our careers. Nevertheless, we often end up spending more hours at work than we do with our families. Having children is a wonderful experience and gives meaning to your life, but they do require a lot of time. My wife and I have five children all under the age of 15. I do not think that we have short-changed them in terms of family time even though Louise and I have had successful careers as physician-scientists. I also do not think that you have to limit the size of your family because you are concerned that you might not have enough time for your career. If anything, having children may cause you to be more efficient in terms of managing your career and family activities. You should not forgo becoming a physician-scientist because you want to have a family. You can have both.

One of the advantages of being a physician-scientist is that you have more "flex time" than full-time clinicians. This makes it easier to attend school events, take kids to the dentist, etc. Another perk of being a physician-scientist is that you may be entitled to take a sabbatical. During your sabbatical year, you will be able to make up for some of the family time that was compromised because of your career. Your sabbatical can offer you the opportunity to do something adventurous and exciting with your family like moving to a new city or country for a year.

When you first start having children, sleep patterns will be compromised. We had five children over the course of seven years. There were long stretches of time when neither of us had adequate sleep. To reduce the burden on both of us, we made an agreement that Louise would be the one who got up at night during the first six months after a child was born. After six months, when they were weaned, I got up to take care of them. We felt that there was no point in both of us getting up and being exhausted the next day when only one parent needed to get up. At the same time, we were both taking call. Despite having many nights with inadequate sleep, both of us still maintained our research productivity. If you are an organized individual with a supportive spouse and a well-organized research team, it is possible to balance career and family.

Many physician-scientists do not start their families until the bulk of their training is finished. During their training, they are used to spending long hours at the hospital and in their laboratories conducting research. This was true in my case. I spent many hours, including evenings and weekends, working on research. When we first started having children, I found that it was harder to spend my evenings and weekends on research. I was able to do extra work only late at night. This is something you must adapt to when your children are born. Later, as your family grows and your children get older, the nature of your family responsibilities changes. You need to be present at your children's after-school activities, attend parent–teacher meetings, help them with their homework, and play with them. As your children get older, their bedtimes get later. As a result, you have less time alone with your spouse and less time to work at night. You have to recognize that at different stages of your career and family life you need to devote different amounts of time to different activities. Recognize these changes and adapt your schedule as needed.

It is important to adapt to the changing requirements of your work and family commitments. Do not compromise family time because of clinical and research requirements. If you do not have enough time in your day to do all of your activities, work late at night as well. If you still do not have enough time, you either do not have enough protected time, are not delegating sufficiently, or are overextended in your research activities.

Additional Issues

Although many of the concerns regarding a physician-scientist career apply fairly equally to men and women, certain issues are more pertinent for one group than the other.

Men in Academic Medicine

In the traditional family structure, the man either solely provided for the family or was the major breadwinner. Today, a male physician-scientist may earn less than his spouse. If the woman earns more money, sometimes the man feels uncomfortable and pressured to earn additional income by consulting or by moonlighting. If this is the case, you need to have a frank discussion with your spouse about this issue. Spending lots of time moonlighting or consulting is sure to impact negatively on your research career and family; unless the extra financial resources are really necessary, taking on these extra commitments is unlikely to be beneficial.

Women in Academic Medicine

I admit that I have limited knowledge about issues relevant to female physician-scientists. Consequently, in writing this section I closely observed and consulted with my wife, Dr. Louise Pilote. Louise is an academic internist and an academic health services researcher with an MPH and a PhD in epidemiology. She is also Chief of the Division of General Internal Medicine at McGill and is the mother of our five children.

Until recently, most physician-scientists were men. That situation is changing rapidly. Close to 50% of students now admitted to medical school are women. As a result, over the next few decades, we will likely see that half of the new physician-scientists will be women. Currently, however, due to the smaller number of female physician-scientists, women may find themselves faced with greater challenges than men. Women may receive little encouragement. They may be told that it is difficult for women to succeed as physician-scientists. In addition, there are fewer role models for women physician-scientists. Until recently, many women who entered the profession of medicine became full-time clinicians rather than physician-scientists. There is a relative dearth of female physician-scientists to have as mentors. Women are also less likely to enter MD-PhD programs. As a result, aspiring female physician-scientists meet few successful female physician-scientists who can guide them on the pathway. Also, many women feel that they have to be better than their male counterparts to be considered equal, and they worry that they will not be able to "super compete" at more advanced levels.

In addition to these concerns, female physician-scientists often have a harder time balancing their careers and family than male physician-scientists. Women have all the same career pressures as men, but they often have an extraordinary amount of family responsibilities as well. In most families, even when both the husband and wife are working, the division of labor is still not egalitarian. The wife still often performs the bulk of the family responsibilities, even though she has a full-time career as a physician-scientist. Besides clinical responsibilities, research responsibilities, teaching responsibilities, and administrative responsibilities, female physician-scientists often come home to major childcare and household responsibilities. In a traditional household, the bulk of the cooking and cleaning is still done by the wife. This situation is far from ideal. It is not possible to be a do-it-all homemaker and a maximally productive physician-scientist.

A major issue for female physician-scientists is that sometimes, particularly at the beginning of their careers, they believe that they have to do it all. They want to be excellent physician-scientists as well as do-it-all homemakers. Unfortunately, there are not enough hours in the day to accomplish both of these goals. It is important that you delegate as many mundane household tasks as possible to reserve your home time for quality time with your children and spouse.

One of the issues that my wife was concerned about when we first started having children was that she was not being a good mother. She felt that perhaps she should stay at home full-time to devote all of her time to our children. After each birth, she spent three–six months at home. Although she did not do any clinical activities during that time, she maintained her research program through e-mail, telephone conferences, and biweekly visits to the hospital. As soon as maternity leave was over, she went back to work full-time. She was able to maintain her research program while taking time off to be with the children, and when she went back to work full-time, she continued to work hard to spend as much time as possible with the children. Many of her concerns were alleviated as she realized that we were able to successfully maintain our research careers without short-changing our family lives. In addition, we both believe it is very positive for our children to see their mother as a role model. When they see that she is a responsible, intelligent physician, researcher, mother and spouse, they can be proud. Our children see that my wife is contributing to society and the creation of knowledge. Louise and I are happy to be able to set this example for our children.

Solutions for many of the above issues are evolving. The present culture is changing to account for the growing prevalence of female physician-scientists. Women are increasingly being recruited for senior faculty positions in addition to key leadership roles in the administration of research institutions. Institutions are becoming more cognizant of the presence of female physician-scientists. Innovative solutions are being implemented to provide shorter working hours, more flexible schedules, and daycares located in hospitals and research centers. However, female physician-scientists still have an unusually difficult position. It is harder for them to balance the role of career and family. Nevertheless, there are many female physician-scientists who have done it successfully. If you are considering becoming a physician-scientist but are worried about these issues, speak with female physician-scientists who have been successful.

Outside Activities

In addition to making time for your career and family, it is also important to make time for you. You may enjoy being involved in other activities or just spending some "alone time" reading or going for a walk. This can be difficult to work into your schedule, but if you are creative, there are ways you can make it work. For example, everyone should be involved in regular physical activity. If you can find no time to go to the gym, try exercising at home. In our house, we have a Stairmaster, an exercise ball, and free weights. For my birthday, my wife arranged for a personal trainer to come to our house. The trainer comes to the house every other week in one evening after dinner and homework. Exercising at home saves me a lot of time. My wife also exercises with the personal trainer on alternate weeks.

There are many other activities in which you can become involved. Everyone has his or her own interests. If you are an active physician-scientist and you have a family, you will have limited time to be involved in these activities. Choose one or two that are high-priority for you, whether it is volunteering, religious activities, going to a country house on weekends, or playing a musical instrument. Whatever your interests are, be systematic in pursuing them in tandem with your career and family activities. If you want anything to happen, you must actively make time for it and build it into your schedule or it will not come to pass.

Summary

Balancing your research activities, your clinical activities, and your family life can be the single most difficult issue you face as a physician-scientist. It is a constant juggling act. It often takes years to achieve the proper balance. It is important to recognize that other physician-scientists have successfully balanced career and family life. Speak with them about how they did it. There are multiple strategies that can help. The most important is that you get professional help so that you can delegate some of the non-quality time activities at home. You also need to have open and frank discussions with your spouse and your children; they need to help you. Prioritize your activities and be very organized about planning and managing the time you spend on each activity. Finally, delegate as much of your non-creative research work as possible so that you can concentrate your limited time on high-value activities. If you are an organized and determined individual, you can be very productive as a physician-scientist and still have a warm and healthy home life.

Key Points

- Spend time early in your career establishing your research program.
- Create "protected time" for your family.
- Delegate non-creative research work to coordinators, assistants, and secretaries.
- Delegate household chores to a housekeeper and routine childcare to a nanny.
- Divide responsibilities among family members so no one is overburdened.
- Make time for physical activities and hobbies.
- If you are overextended, delegate, reduce the scope of your activities, and negotiate more protected time.
- Discuss with senior colleagues how they manage all their activities.
- Be organized and designate time for specific activities.

Suggested Readings

1. Carnes M. Balancing family and career: advice from the trenches. Ann Intern Med 1996; 125: 618–620.
2. Carr PL, Ash AS, Friedman RH, et al. Relation of family responsibilities and gender to the productivity and career satisfaction of medical faculty. Ann Intern Med 1998; 129: 532–538.
3. Harris JP, Ariessohn ML. Economic, family, and length-of-training issues that influence the selection of a clinician-scientist career path in otolaryngology. Otolaryngol Head Neck Surg 2008; 139: 100–104.
4. Levinson W, Kaufman K, Tolle SW. Women in academic medicine: strategies for balancing career and personal life. J Am Med Womens Assoc 1992; 47: 25–28.
5. Linzer M. Preventing burnout in academic medicine. Arch Intern Med 2009; 169: 927–928.
6. McHenry CR. In search of balance: a successful career, health, and family. Am J Surg 2007; 193: 293–297.
7. Rubin DC. Balancing family and career: addressing the challenges facing dual-career couples. Gastrointest Endosc 2006; 63: 831–833.
8. Seal DW. Child planning required: a father's perspective on balancing career and family within academic psychiatry. Acad Psychiatry 2007; 31: 143–145.
9. Shanafelt TD, West CP, Sloan JA, et al. Career fit and burnout among academic faculty. Arch Intern Med 2009; 169: 990–995.
10. Verlander G. Female physicians: balancing career and family. Acad Psychiatry 2004; 28: 331–336.

Chapter 19
Improving the Physician-Scientist Pathway

*You are doing your best only when you are trying to improve
what you are doing.*

–Unknown

Introduction

As you become a senior physician-scientist, your role will increasingly involve
mentorship, management of large research teams, and directing large research programs. You should become increasingly involved in transferring the knowledge you
have acquired to junior physician-scientists. At the same time, your institution may
enlist you to help improve the physician-scientist pathway at your medical center. The two main issues that most academic medical centers need to improve with
respect to the physician-scientist pathway are recruitment and retention. How can
we increase the number of individuals entering this pathway? How can we keep
individuals from dropping out once they are in the pathway? Both issues are critical.
If we want to maintain and strengthen the physician-scientist pathway, we have to
develop interventions that address these two issues. To gain insights into the obstacles associated with the physician-scientist pathway, my research team surveyed
a group of 16 individuals involved in the physician-scientist pathway at McGill
University. In this chapter, I discuss some of the obstacles we identified, as well
as several potential interventions.

Survey of Physician-Scientists

We conducted semi-structured interviews with 16 individuals involved in the
physician-scientist pathway at McGill University. The individuals ranged from
fellows who were just becoming physician-scientists, to mid-career and senior
physician-scientists. We also surveyed the director of the research institute at
one of the McGill hospitals. The individuals worked at four different hospitals
and represented multiple clinical areas, including cardiology, endocrinology, general internal medicine, hematology, obstetrics/gynecology, and orthopedic surgery.

M.J. Eisenberg, *The Physician Scientist's Career Guide*,
DOI 10.1007/978-1-60327-908-6_19, © Springer Science+Business Media, LLC 2011

Several issues were commonly identified by these individuals as obstacles for physician-scientists (Table 19.1).

First, it is difficult for an established physician to find time to obtain the training necessary to become a successful physician-scientist. Most physician-scientists we interviewed became interested in this career pathway as medical students. Many pointed out that, to increase the number of physician-scientists, medical schools need to identify promising medical students and get more of them involved in research. Identifying physicians who are already in fellowship or junior faculty positions and turning them into physician-scientists is unlikely to be successful.

Table 19.1 Survey of 16 individuals involved in the physician-scientist pathway

What is the one measure that should be taken to increase the number of physician-scientists?
- Create financial incentives
- Create physician-scientist tracks during residency
- Increase opportunities for continued funding of research
- Increase funding opportunities for research training during and after residency

What is the one measure that could decrease the failure rate among physician-scientists?
- Sufficient protected time
- Increased opportunities for continued funding of research
- One-to-one mentorship with senior physician-scientists
- Financial incentives

What is the single most important obstacle to success as a physician-scientist?
- Lack of opportunities for collaboration while developing his/her career
- Trying to balance research, clinical duties, and life outside of work
- Lack of support by an environment insensitive to the tools required for success
- Clinical responsibilities that interrupt research

What are the character traits that a physician-scientist should possess to be successful?
- Persistence and determination in the face of failure
- Ability to accept criticism
- Curiosity
- Ability to remain highly focused on a question or problem
- Willing to take risks

Does a significant disparity exist between the career income potential of a physician-scientist *vs.* that of a full-time physician? Does it matter?
- Huge difference between researcher and clinician
- Yes, there is a disparity, but it does not matter
- It matters a great deal: Career insecurity (scholarships, tenure, etc.) *versus* the ease of making a good living practicing the medical art is a fatal distraction for many

Assuming the status quo is maintained, would you recommend aspiring physicians/researchers to become physician-scientist? Why or why not?
- Yes, because the challenge of discovery and the gratification thereof is unique
- Probably not. Most aspiring physician-scientists do not have the drive or willingness to accept the financial sacrifices
- Yes. The opportunity to meet the best and the brightest, and constantly learn and be challenged, render tolerable the sacrifices of time with family, frustrations of scarce funding and the difficulties of publication

Second, the difficulty in obtaining grants was identified as being one of the major obstacles to success, particularly at the junior faculty level. The pervasive feeling was that it is very difficult for new physician-scientists to be competitive at the national level. A possible solution suggested was to substantially increase the number of small internal grants available to junior faculty members. Small internal grants allow junior faculty members to generate pilot data, making their grant proposals more competitive at the national level.

Third, mentoring was raised as an important issue by virtually all individuals interviewed. They noted a lack of formal mentoring at all career levels, including medical student, residency, fellowship, and junior faculty levels. Especially at the medical student level, they felt that a mentor can play a critical role in getting the individual interested in research. If medical students have poor research experiences at the onset, it is unlikely they will be attracted to this career path. The physician-scientists suggested introducing a more formal mentoring process. They made the point that, even at the junior faculty level, mentoring is very important. Many new physician-scientists have never seen or written a grant. As a result, it is difficult for them to be competitive unless they have formal input from more senior physician-scientists.

A fourth commonly identified issue was that of protected time for research. It was agreed that protected time is critical for junior faculty members to succeed as physician-scientists. Although physician-scientists are promised protected time at the beginning of their careers, it is often encroached upon. Most funding agencies that provide career awards mandate that at least 50% of a physician-scientist's time be devoted to research. However, the amount of salary support provided to individual researchers may cover only a fraction of their salaries. As a result, pressure is often placed on the individual by the division head to do more clinical work to justify their salaries. At the beginning of a physician-scientist's career, it is unlikely that they will be successful if they do not have adequate protected time. Therefore, protected time needs to be more than a phrase; it needs to be an idea that all division and department heads are committed to.

Our survey was not an exhaustive study. Nevertheless, it was helpful in clarifying some of the issues that are obstacles to success. The information generated was also helpful in providing ideas about potential interventions that could strengthen the physician-scientist pathway.

System-Level Changes

System-level changes are needed for many of these issues to be resolved. Historically, physician-scientists who trained at leading academic medical centers went on to become successful researchers, as well as division chiefs and department heads at other universities. This paradigm is less and less the case. Because of funding cuts, there has been an increasing need to justify salaries. Consequently, there is less emphasis on performing research, and the commitment to research at some academic medical centers has become much weaker. The systems at these medical centers need to be rejuvenated, so that division and department heads are firmly committed to producing academic physicians who will become successful physician-scientists. Research needs to be encouraged at every level of the academic medical center.

Experiences as Director of Clinical Research for the McGill Cardiology Fellowship Program

Research is a mandated aspect of training for cardiology fellows at McGill University. However, as Director for Clinical Research for the cardiology training program, I know that relatively few of our fellows manage to complete a research project during their training. Our fellows have four months of protected time for research during their training, yet fewer than 50% manage to complete a research project and even fewer manage to publish an article.

To improve this situation, when individuals interview for training positions, they should be advised that research is a critical component of the fellowship. Research experience is important, even for those who intend to be pure clinicians. Exposure to research is valuable when it comes to reading the medical literature. In an academic training program, there should be an emphasis on recruiting fellows who have demonstrated an interest in and an aptitude for research. It should be mandated by the program (and enforced by the program director) that fellows complete a research project and produce a manuscript suitable for submission to a journal prior to finishing their fellowship. Both the training program director and the division chief need to be firmly committed to the concept that each trainee needs adequate research experience. Trainees cannot have sufficient research experience unless they are committed to completing a research project and writing a manuscript prior to finishing their training.

In addition to investing the research and clinical components of the fellowship with equal importance, it would be useful to increase the time spent on research during both medical school and residency. Residents and fellows should also be encouraged to seek additional formal research training that will give them the skills to function as independent researchers. Many fellowships now expect trainees to obtain Master's degrees in a research discipline as part of their program.

Potential Interventions

Many potential interventions can be used to increase the number of individuals attracted to a career as a physician-scientist and decrease the attrition rate among beginning physician-scientists. Some of these interventions are described below.

Formal Mentorship Program

A formal mentorship program for medical students, residents, fellows, and particularly junior faculty members can be introduced. For example, many medical students receive scholarships to do summer research projects. There could be formal meetings for these students where they meet with faculty members and discuss a career as a physician-scientist. Although each of these students is assigned a research supervisor, there is often no formalized discussion on how the student can pursue a research career. The ideal time to discuss this issue is in the summer when most medical students are physically present in laboratories. In addition, residents, fellows, and new physician-scientists should be assigned formal research mentors. Although formally matching up a trainee with a mentor will not work in all situations, it will at least establish a dialogue.

Mandatory Grant Review

One of the major obstacles to success for junior physician-scientists is the difficulty in obtaining operating grants. It is hard to be competitive at the national level when you have never seen or written a grant. I sit on several grant review committees, and when I review an application from a junior faculty member, I often notice that the grant application could have been substantially improved if there had been a formalized review process at the applicant's hospital prior to submission. Some hospitals have a formalized review process where junior faculty members cannot submit grants to funding agencies until faculty members with more experience have reviewed them. Some institutions even require reviews of senior faculty grant proposals as well. Having a mandatory review mechanism for grants of junior faculty members could substantially improve the quality of the applications submitted, thereby increasing the chances of these individuals receiving funding and ultimately building successful research careers.

Internal Awards for Junior Faculty

Many academic medical centers have only a small number of internal awards available for junior physician-scientists. When I review grants from junior faculty members at some institutions, I often observe that the applicant has received several small internal awards that enabled them to do some pilot work. These grants significantly enhance the application. The funding allows the junior faculty member to hire a research assistant and perform some pilot work, and it provides credibility to both the researcher and the project. Pilot study data are important when applying to a national funding agency for grant support. Additionally, comments received from internal competitions can be very helpful in improving the grant before submitting it externally. As a result, increasing the number of small, internal operating awards could substantially enhance the physician-scientist pathway.

Research Design and Methodology Course

A summer course in research design and methodology can help research trainees and junior faculty members prepare research protocols. I participated in such a course when I was a research fellow at the Cardiovascular Research Institute of the University of California at San Francisco. The course took place during the summer after the new research fellows had arrived. Each week, we reviewed different epidemiologic principles, and we were responsible for the preparation of a study protocol by the end of the summer. A research design and methodology course would also allow individuals interested in research to learn some fundamental research principles and to collaborate on improving their research protocols. Because the deadlines for many grant competitions are in September or October, a summer course like this can be helpful to research fellows and junior faculty members.

Biomedical Writing Course

A course in biomedical writing should be available to all research trainees and junior physician-scientists and should also be made available to medical students, residents, and fellows. These courses can significantly improve the quality of an individual's biomedical writing and grant applications. In addition, it gives individuals with minimal experience at biomedical writing the chance to get their hands wet. A positive experience in a biomedical writing course can help attract and retain individuals to the physician-scientist pathway.

Summer Course for High School and University Students

Many high school and university students conduct research during the summer at academic medical centers. These students are often isolated in various laboratories and have little contact with other students and other individuals interested in research careers. They could attend meetings to learn about careers in biomedical research. These meetings could provide them with the opportunity to present their research projects and obtain feedback from groups outside their laboratory. Exposure to a variety of successful physician-scientists would enhance the likelihood of these students being attracted to the physician-scientist pathway.

Seminar for Physician-Scientists

Many years ago, my hospital introduced a monthly seminar for physician-scientists. It was unsuccessful and was ultimately abandoned. The reason it was unsuccessful was that when we met once a month, we would take turns presenting our research projects to each other. However, each physician-scientist was in a different field, and much of the time, we could not follow the details of each other's research. Although we were all physician-scientists, we did not have much in common with respect to our areas of research and the methodologies used. Some did basic science research, some did translational research, some did clinical research, and some did population research.

However, there might be room for a seminar of a different kind; a seminar that focused on the process rather than the substance of being a physician-scientist. Participants would discuss ways to improve the chances of success for junior physician-scientists. Specific topics could include grantsmanship, biomedical writing, and how to build a research team. A meeting of this kind, focused more on the process of succeeding as a physician-scientist rather than on the substance, might be more useful than one that focuses purely on science.

Improving the Physician-Scientist Pathway: The Steering Committee

If you are considering improving the physician-scientist pathway at your institution, determine the key people who need to be involved. Consider putting together a steering committee to address obstacles to the physician-scientist pathway. This committee could include individuals at different stages of their careers. They could cover the spectrum of the physician-scientist pathway, from those who are just entering the pathway such as clinical and research fellows, to those who are new investigators, to those who are mid-career and senior investigators. Some of the individuals represented might include:

1. Individuals at the faculty development office.
2. University/academic department chiefs.
3. Head of the research institute.
4. Director of the clinical investigator program (if one exists).
5. Division heads.
6. Training program directors.
7. Deputy directors of research (e.g., basic science, clinical).
8. Executive administrators at the research institute.
9. Director of Clinical Epidemiology.
10. Junior, mid-career, and senior physician-scientists.
11. Physician-scientists with a spectrum of research interests (basic science, translational, clinical, and population).
12. Physician-scientists with international experience and stature.
13. Research fellows and graduate students.

Summary

Interventions at the institutional level can help attract and retain more individuals to the physician-scientist career. As a consequence, the quantity and quality of biomedical research will increase, and improved health for individuals and for the population will result. For physicians who do not become physician-scientists, greater exposure to research during training will give them a better appreciation for how research is conducted. This experience will help them better understand the journal articles that they will be reading for the rest of their careers. Ultimately, clinical practice will improve, because individuals exposed to the research process are much more evidence-based in their interpretation and application of the medical literature. During our early careers as physician-scientists, many of us narrowly focus on our own areas of research. As we become senior physician-scientists, we should consider how to give back to the system, how to help recruit more potential physician-scientists, and how to help the current crop of junior physician-scientists establish successful careers.

Key Points

- Introduce interventions to increase the number of individuals entering the physician-scientist path.
- Introduce interventions to reduce the number of dropouts from the pathway.
- Provide training in all elements of research, so that new junior faculty members are able to set up laboratories, prepare grants, and lead their own research teams.
- Reinforce research as a critical component of clinical training programs.
- Introduce a formal mentorship program at all levels of training.
- Introduce a mandatory review of junior faculty grants by senior faculty before submission to funding agencies.
- Increase the number of internal awards for junior faculty to improve their chances of obtaining peer-reviewed funding.
- Encourage your institution to develop research methodology courses, biomedical writing courses, and ongoing seminars.

Suggested Reading

1. Donath E, Filion KB, Eisenberg MJ. Improving the Clinician-Scientist pathway: a survey of Clinician-Scientists. Arch Intern Med 2009; 169: 1242–1244.
2. Hauser SL, McArthur JC. Saving the clinician-scientist: report of the ANA long range planning committee. Ann Neurol 2006; 60: 278–285.
3. Krebsbach PH, Ignelzi MA Jr. Failure to attract and retain clinician/scientist faculty puts our profession at risk. J Dent Res 1999; 78: 1576–1578.
4. Lemoine NR. The clinician-scientist: a rare breed under threat in a hostile environment. Dis Model Mech 2008; 1: 12–14.
5. McKelvie J, McGhee CN. The clinician scientist-quo vadis? Clin Exp Ophthalmol 2009; 37: 247–248.
6. Schrier RW. Ensuring the survival of the clinician-scientist. Acad Med 1997; 72: 589–594.

Chapter 20
Concluding Remarks

Success is a journey, not a destination.

–Ben Sweetland

In this book, I have tried to relate some of the knowledge I acquired over the past two decades as a physician-scientist. To succeed as a physician-scientist, you need to develop a wide knowledge base and a variety of skills. Most of this knowledge and the majority of these skills can only be acquired experientially. They are very difficult to obtain in an organized and formal fashion. I hope that over the few hours you spent reading this book, you have become familiar with some of the knowledge and skills that you will require to be successful as a physician-scientist. I recognize that I have not talked much about the love of science and the love of discovery: rather, I focused on concrete issues like how to write an original research article, how to obtain grant support, and how to lecture effectively. If you have read this book, it is quite likely that you are already committed to the development of new knowledge and that you love science and inquiry. It is my hope that reading this book will make it easier for you to succeed as a physician-scientist.

I would like to conclude by recounting an event that happened several years ago. This event illustrates why we need physician-scientists and the importance of contributions that physician-scientists make.

Several years ago, at the age of 44, my brother suffered a cardiac arrest. He was a pediatrician with a wife and seven children. He had a history of mitral valve prolapse and frequent premature ventricular contractions but was otherwise well. One morning, he suddenly collapsed. Thankfully, he was with a teenager who knew CPR and immediately began chest compressions. Bystanders called 911, and an ambulance quickly arrived. He was shocked multiple times, intubated, and then transported to the University of Rochester Medical Center, where both of us were born and where I went to medical school. He was transferred to the cardiac catheterization laboratory, where coronary and cerebral angiographies were performed. Both were normal. He also underwent a left ventriculogram that showed an ejection fraction of less than 20%.

He was then transferred to the intensive care unit where he spent the next 3 days in a coma. He was treated for the first 24 h with therapeutic hypothermia. He required ventilator support, vasopressors, and cardioversion for transient atrial fibrillation. After 3 days, he woke up and was extubated. He managed to walk to the step-down unit where he remained for several more days. He had a defibrillator implanted and was discharged from the hospital. His left ventricular ejection fraction subsequently returned to normal. Within several months he was back at work as a pediatrician, with no cognitive dysfunction. Every year, he celebrates the anniversary of his survival with his family and friends.

I think frequently about what happened to my brother. It is clear to me that had he suffered a cardiac arrest 40 or 50 years ago, he would have died. Over just a few decades, physician-scientists have developed new diagnostic techniques, therapeutic approaches, drugs, and technologies, all of which contributed to my brother's survival. From the development of cardiopulmonary resuscitation to the development of defibrillation, and from the development of technology used for artificial ventilation to the performance of clinical trials that demonstrated the value of therapeutic hypothermia, physician-scientists have slowly built up the knowledge and skills required to save many lives; lives that would otherwise be lost. No device, procedure, or therapy was developed by a single physician-scientist alone. Rather, it was many physician-scientists over many years that developed and refined each individual component that was essential to my brother's survival. Importantly, many of the individuals who took care of my brother in the hospital were trained by physician-scientists or were physician-scientists themselves. These individuals helped develop and continue to practice the evidence-based medicine that was essential to my brother's survival.

My point in relating this story is that physician-scientists really do make a difference in the world. There is great satisfaction in knowing that you have contributed to the survival and quality of life of so many individuals. Although you may not realize it in your day-to-day activities, you are contributing to the discovery of new knowledge that will improve patient care for decades to come. Finally, you are also training the next generation of individuals who will extend our current knowledge base even further. I highly recommend this career path to you. There are few career paths that are so rewarding and meaningful.

Appendices

The cure for boredom is curiosity. There is no cure for curiosity.

–Dorothy Parker

Appendix 1: MD–PhD Programs in the United States

School name	Location	Website
University of Alabama School of Medicine	Birmingham, AL	http://www.uasom.uab.edu/mdphd/
University of South Alabama College of Medicine	Mobile, AL	http://www.southalabama.edu/com/phd.shtml
University of Arizona Health Sciences Center	Tucson, AZ	http://www.medicine.arizona.edu/mdphd/
University of Arkansas College of Medicine	Little Rock, AR	http://www.uams.edu/mdphd/
Loma Linda University School of Medicine	Loma Linda, CA	http://www.llu.edu/llu/medicine/basicsciences/msp.html
Stanford University School of Medicine	Stanford, CA	http://mstp.stanford.edu/
University of California, Davis School of Medicine	Davis, CA	http://www.ucdmc.ucdavis.edu/mdphd/
University of California, Irvine School of Medicine	Irvine, CA	http://www.ucihs.uci.edu/mdphd/
University of California, Los Angeles School of Medicine	Los Angeles, CA	http://www.medsch.ucla.edu/mstp/
University of California, San Diego School of Medicine	San Diego, CA	http://meded.ucsd.edu/asa/mstp/
University of California, San Francisco School of Medicine	San Francisco, CA	http://medschool.ucsf.edu/mstp/
University of Southern California School of Medicine	Los Angeles, CA	http://www.usc.edu/schools/medicine/education/degrees_programs/mdp/mdphd.html
University of Colorado	Denver, CO	http://www.uchsc.edu/som/mstp/index.html

(continued)

M.J. Eisenberg, *The Physician Scientist's Career Guide*,
DOI 10.1007/978-1-60327-908-6, © Springer Science+Business Media, LLC 2011

School name	Location	Website
University of Connecticut School of Medicine	Farmington, CT	http://medicine.uchc.edu/index.html
Yale University School of Medicine	New Haven, CT	http://info.med.yale.edu/mdphd/program/index.html
Georgetown University Medical Center	Washington, DC	http://biomedgrad.georgetown.edu/MDPhD/index.html
George Washington University Medical Center	Washington, DC	http://www.gwumc.edu/edu/admis/html/academics/mdphd.html
Howard University College of Medicine	Washington, DC	http://medicine.howard.edu/education/programs/degrees.htm
University of Florida College of Medicine	Gainesville, FL	http://www.med.ufl.edu/md-phd/
University of Miami Miller School of Medicine	Miami, FL	http://chroma.med.miami.edu/mdphd/
University of South Florida College of Medicine	Tampa, FL	http://health.usf.edu/medicine/graduate studies/index.htm
Emory University School of Medicine	Atlanta, GA	http://www.med.emory.edu/education/MDPHD/
Medical College of Georgia	Augusta, GA	http://www.mcg.edu/som/mdphd/index.htm
Loyola University of Chicago Stritch School of Medicine	Maywood, IL	http://www.stritch.luc.edu/node/83
Northwestern University Feinberg School of Medicine	Chicago, IL	http://mstp.northwestern.edu/
Rosalind Franklin University of Medicine and Science	North Chicago, IL	http://www.rosalindfranklin.edu/dnn/sgps/hidden/SGPS/MDPhD/tabid/710/Default.aspx
University of Chicago Pritzker School of Medicine	Chicago, IL	http://pritzker.bsd.uchicago.edu/joint degrees/combined/mdphd.shtml
University of Illinois College of Medicine at Chicago	Chicago, IL	http://chicago.medicine.uic.edu/mstp
University of Illinois at Urbana-Champaign College of Medicine	Urbana, IL	http://www.med.uiuc.edu/msp/
Indiana University School of Medicine	Indianapolis, IN	http://grad.medicine.iu.edu/body.cfm?id=1851
University of Iowa Carver College of Medicine	Iowa City, IA	http://www.medicine.uiowa.edu/mstp/
University of Kansas Medical Center	Kansas City, KS	http://www3.kumc.edu/mdphd/
University of Kentucky College of Medicine	Lexington, KY	http://www.mc.uky.edu/mdphd/
University of Louisville School of Medicine	Louisville, KY	http://louisville.edu/medschool/mdphd
Louisiana State University School of Medicine	New Orleans, LA	http://www.medschool.lsuhsc.edu/admissions/programs.aspx#MD
Louisiana State University, Health Sciences Center	Shreveport, LA	http://www.sh.lsuhsc.edu/index.html

(continued)

School name	Location	Website
Tulane University School of Medicine	New Orleans, LA	http://www.biomedicalsciences.tulane.edu/main.php?page=MD/Ph.D%20Curriculum&navy=7
Johns Hopkins University School of Medicine	Baltimore, MD	http://www.hopkinsmedicine.org/mdphd/
National Institutes of Health Graduate Partnerships Program	Bethesda, MD	http://gpp.nih.gov/
Uniformed Services University of the Health Sciences	Bethesda, MD	http://www.usuhs.mil/index.html
University of Maryland School of Medicine	Baltimore, MD	http://mdphd.umaryland.edu/
Boston University School of Medicine	Boston, MA	http://www.bumc.bu.edu/mdphd/
Harvard Medical School	Boston, MA	http://www.hms.harvard.edu/md_phd/index.html
Tufts University Graduate School of Biomedical Sciences	Boston, MA	http://www.tufts.edu/sackler/programs/combined.html
University of Massachusetts Medical School	Worchester, MA	http://www.umassmed.edu/mdphd/index.aspx
Michigan State University College of Human Medicine	East Lansing, MI	http://mdadmissions.msu.edu/main/mdphd.htm
University of Michigan Medical School	Ann Arbor, MI	http://www.med.umich.edu/medschool/mstp/
Wayne State University School of Medicine	Detroit, MI	http://mdphdprogram.med.wayne.edu/
Mayo Clinic College of Medicine	Rochester, MN	http://www.mayo.edu/mgs/mstp.html
University of Minnesota, Minneapolis School of Medicine	Minneapolis, MN	http://www.med.umn.edu/mdphd/
University of Mississippi School of Medicine	Jackson, MS	http://som.umc.edu/admissions.html#mdphd
Saint Louis University School of Medicine	St. Louis, MO	http://medschool.slu.edu/admissions/index.php?page=mdphd-program
University of Missouri, Columbia School of Medicine	Columbia, MO	http://mdphd.missouri.edu/
Washington University School of Medicine	St. Louis, MO	http://mstp.wustl.edu/
Creighton University School of Medicine	Omaha, NE	http://medschool.creighton.edu/medicine/index.php
University of Nebraska College of Medicine	Omaha, NE	http://www.unmc.edu/dept/brtp/index.cfm?webtype=graphics&L1_ID=8&CONREF=18
University of Nevada School of Medicine	Reno, NV	http://www.medicine.nevada.edu/dept/asa/prospective_applicants/programs_home.htm
Dartmouth Medical School	Hanover, NH	http://dms.dartmouth.edu/admissions/curriculum/mdphd/

(continued)

School name	Location	Website
University of Medicine and Dentistry of New Jersey, School of Biomedical Sciences	Newark, NJ	http://www.umdnj.edu/gsbsnweb/ academic_programs/md_phd.htm
University of Medicine and Dentistry of New Jersey, Robert Wood Johnson Medical School	Piscataway, NJ	http://rwjms.umdnj.edu/education/gsbs/ md_phd_program/index.html
University of New Mexico School of Medicine	Albuquerque, NM	http://hsc.unm.edu/som/research/bsgp/ mdphdwelcome.shtm
Albert Einstein College of Medicine of Yeshiva University	Bronx, NY	http://mstp.aecom.yu.edu/
Columbia University College of Physicians and Surgeons	New York, NY	http://cpmcnet.columbia.edu/dept/mdphd/ home/
Weill/Cornell/Rockefeller/ Sloan-Kettering Tri-institutional Program	New York, NY	http://www.med.cornell.edu/mdphd/
Mount Sinai School of Medicine	New York, NY	http://www.mountsinai.org/Education
New York Medical College	Valhalla, NY	http://www.nymc.edu/gsbms/md-phd-program.asp
New York University School of Medicine	New York, NY	http://mdphd.med.nyu.edu/
SUNY at Buffalo School of Medicine	Buffalo, NY	http://www.smbs.buffalo.edu/rbe/mstp/
SUNY at Stony Brook Health Sciences Center	Stony Brook, NY	http://www.pharm.stonybrook.edu/mstp/ index.html
SUNY Downstate Medical Center College of Medicine	Brooklyn, NY	http://sls.downstate.edu/admissions/ medicine/mdpdh_program.html
SUNY Upstate Medical University	Syracuse, NY	http://www.upstate.edu/com/specialprog. php
University of Rochester School of Medicine	Rochester, NY	http://www.urmc.rochester.edu/smd/mstp/ ?redir=www.urmc.edu
Wake Forest University, Bowman Gray School of Medicine	Winston-Salem, NC	http://www1.wfubmc.edu/mdphd
East Carolina University, Brody School of Medicine	Greenville, NC	http://www.ecu.edu/cs-dhs/med/MD_PhD. cfm
Duke University School of Medicine	Durham, NC	http://www.mstp.duke.edu/
University of North Carolina School of Medicine	Chapel Hill, NC	http://www.med.unc.edu/mdphd/
University of North Dakota School of Medicine and Health Sciences	Grand Forks, ND	http://www.med.und.nodak.edu/mdphd/
Case Western Reserve University School of Medicine	Cleveland, OH	http://mstp.cwru.edu/

(continued)

School name	Location	Website
Ohio State University College of Medicine and Public Health	Columbus, OH	http://www.osumdphd.org/
University of Cincinnati College of Medicine	Cincinnati, OH	http://www.med.uc.edu/pstp/
University of Toledo College of Medicine	Toledo, OH	http://www.utoledo.edu/med/mdphd/index.html
Wright State University Boonshoft School of Medicine	Dayton, OH	http://www.med.wright.edu/md-phd/
University of Oklahoma Health Science Center	Oklahoma City, OK	http://mdphd.ouhsc.edu/
Oregon Health and Science University School of Medicine	Portland, OR	http://www.ohsu.edu/mdphd/
Drexel University College of Medicine	Philadelphia, PA	http://www.drexelmed.edu/Home/Admissions/MDProgram/DualDegrees.aspx
Jefferson Medical College	Philadelphia, PA	http://www.jefferson.edu/jmc/admissions/05_JMC_prospectus.pdf
Penn State University College of Medicine	Hershey, PA	http://www.pennstatehershey.org/web/mdphd/home
University of Pennsylvania School of Medicine	Philadelphia, PA	http://www.med.upenn.edu/mstp/program.shtml
University of Pittsburgh & Carnegie Mellon University	Pittsburgh, PA	https://www.mdphd.pitt.edu/
Temple University School of Medicine	Philadelphia, PA	http://www.temple.edu/medicine/education/dualdegree/mdphd.htm
Brown University Alpert Medical School	Providence, RI	http://bms.brown.edu/mdphd/
Medical University of South Carolina	Charleston, SC	http://www.musc.edu/grad/mstp/index.html
University of South Carolina School of Medicine	Columbia, SC	http://pathmicro.med.sc.edu/graduate/md-phd.htm
University of South Dakota Sanford School of Medicine	Vermillion, SD	http://www.usd.edu/med/
Meharry Medical College School of Medicine	Nashville, TN	http://www.mmc.edu
University of Tennessee Health Science Center	Memphis, TN	http://www.utmem.edu/Medicine/Admissions/index.php?doc=./inc/PROSPECTIVE_MDPHD.htm
Vanderbilt University School of Medicine	Nashville, TN	https://medschool.mc.vanderbilt.edu/mstp/
Baylor College of Medicine	Houston, TX	http://www.bcm.edu/mstp/
Texas A & M University Health Sciences Center	College Station, TX	http://medicine.tamhsc.edu/education/md-phd/index.html
Texas Tech University Health Science Center	Lubbock, TX	http://www.ttuhsc.edu/gsbs/academics/MDPhDProgram.aspx
University of Texas, Medical Branch at Galveston	Galveston, TX	http://www.utmb.edu/mdphd/

(continued)

School name	Location	Website
University of Texas Health Science Center at Houston	Houston, TX	http://www.uth.tmc.edu/gsbs/programs/mdphd/index.html
University of Texas, San Antonio Medical School	San Antonio, TX	http://som.uthscsa.edu/Admissions/MDPhD.asp
University of Texas, Southwestern Medical Center	Dallas, TX	http://www.utsouthwestern.edu/graduate school/mstp.html
University of Utah School of Medicine	Salt Lake City, UT	http://medicine.utah.edu/mdphd/
University of Vermont College of Medicine	Burlington, VT	http://www.med.uvm.edu/mdphd/TB1+I+C+RL.asp?SiteAreaID=513
Eastern Virginia Medical School	Norfolk, VA	http://www.evms.edu/education/joint-md-mph.html
Virginia Commonwealth University School of Medicine	Richmond, VA	http://www.medschool.vcu.edu/mdphd/
University of Virginia School of Medicine	Charlottesville, VA	http://www.healthsystem.virginia.edu/internet/mstp/mstpprog.cfm
University of Washington School of Medicine	Seattle, WA	http://www.mstp.washington.edu/
West Virginia University School of Medicine	Morgantown, WV	http://www.hsc.wvu.edu/som/resoff/gradprograms/mdphd.asp
Medical College of Wisconsin	Milwaukee, WI	http://www.mcw.edu/display/docid27193.htm
University of Wisconsin Medical School	Madison, WI	http://mstp.med.wisc.edu/

Resources

1. Association of American Medical Colleges. MD-PhD Dual Degree Training. http://www.aamc.org/students/considering/research/mdphd/start.htm. Accessed March 27, 2009.

Appendix 2: MD–PhD Programs in Canada

School name	Location	Website
University of Alberta Faculty of Medicine and Dentistry	Edmonton, AB	http://www.med.ualberta.ca/Home/Education/ MScPhD/mdphd.cfm
University of Calgary Faculty of Medicine	Calgary, AB	http://medicine.ucalgary.ca/grad/programs #MDLM
University of British Columbia Faculty of Medicine	Vancouver, BC	http://www.med.ubc.ca/education/md_ugrad/ mdphd.htm
University of Manitoba Faculty of Medicine	Winnipeg, MB	http://umanitoba.ca/faculties/medicine/units/ physiology/phd.html
Memorial University Faculty of Medicine	St. John's, NL	http://www.med.mun.ca/medicine/home.aspx
Dalhousie University Department of Pharmacology	Halifax, NS	http://pharmacology.medicine.dal.ca/graduate/ mdphd.cfm
McMaster University Faculty of Health Sciences	Hamilton, ON	http://fhs.mcmaster.ca/grad/medsci/MDPHD% 20index.htm
University of Toronto Faculty of Medicine	Toronto, ON	http://www.gradschool.utoronto.ca/programs/ doctoral/MDPhD.htm
University of Western Ontario	London, ON	http://www.schulich.uwo.ca/medicine/md_phd/
McGill University Faculty of Medicine	Montreal, QC	http://www.mcgill.ca/files/medicine/Brochure_ Med-R_2007-08_en.pdf
Université Laval Faculté de Médecine	Quebec City, QC	http://w3.fmed.ulaval.ca/site_fac/
Université de Montréal Faculté de Médecine	Montreal, QC	http://www.med.umontreal.ca/
Université de Sherbrooke Faculté de Médecine	Sherbrooke, QC	http://www.usherbrooke.ca/accueil/english/
University of Saskatchewan College of Medicine	Saskatoon, SK	http://www.medicine.usask.ca/research/ CombinedHandbook.pdf

Resources

1. Association of American Medical Colleges. MD-PhD Dual Degree Training. http://www. aamc.org/students/considering/research/mdphd/start.htm. Accessed March 27, 2009.

Appendix 3a: National Institutes of Health (NIH) – Research Grants (R Series)

Name		Description
R01	Research Project Grant Program	• Most commonly used NIH program • Used to support a specified project, generally for three–five years
R03	Small Grant Program	• Pilot studies, preliminary data collection, secondary analysis of existing data, etc. • Two years, up to $50,000/year • Non-renewable
R13	Conferences & Scientific Meetings	• High-quality conferences that are relevant to NIH's mission • Up to five years, amounts vary
R15	Academic Research Enhancement Award	• Small projects in biomedical and behavioral sciences • Students and faculty in health professional schools • Up to three years, $150,000 total
R21	Exploratory/Developmental Research Grant Award	• Project development, pilot or feasibility studies of exploratory/developmental research • Up to two years, $275,000 total
R24	Resource-Related Research Projects	• Provide resources for problems where multiple expertise is needed to focus on a complex biomedical resource problem • Enhancement of research infrastructure
R25	Education Projects	• Promote interest in, provide training for biomedical research • Develop ways to disseminate scientific discovery into public health and community
R34	Clinical Trial Planning Grant	• For early peer review of the rationale for proposed trials • To support development of elements of clinical trials • One–three years, usually up to $100,000, sometimes up to $450,000
R41/R42	Small Business Technology Transfer	• Stimulate scientific and technological innovation • Cooperative research between small business concerns and research institutions • Up to three years, $850,000 total

(continued)

Name		Description
R43/R44	Small Business Innovative Research	• Stimulate technological research in the private sector • Support ideas of for-profit organizations which have potential for commercialization • Up to three years, $850,000
R56	High Priority, Short-term Project Award	• High priority new or competing renewal R01 applications that fall outside the funding limits of NIH institutions
U01	Research Project Cooperative Agreement	• Specified research projects in an area representing investigator's specific interests and competencies • Substantial involvement anticipated between the awarding Institute and Center • No specific dollar limit
K99/R00	Pathway to Independence Award	• Up to five years of support for promising, post-doctoral research scientists • One–two years mentored support; three years of independent support contingent on securing an independent research position

Appendix 3b: National Institutes of Health (NIH) – Career Development Awards (K Series)

Name	Description
K01 Mentored Research Scientist Development Award	• Support and protected time for supervised career development leading to research independence • Biomedical, behavioral, or clinical sciences • Three–five years, not renewable
K02 Independent Scientist Award	• Support for newly independent scientists who demonstrate need for research focus to enhance research career
K05 Senior Scientist Research & Mentorship Award	• Provide protected time to outstanding senior scientists • To allow focus on research and time for mentoring
K07 Academic Career Award	• Support for the introduction or improvement of curricula • To enhance educational or research capacity at the grantee institution
K08 Mentored Clinical Scientist Research Career Development Award	• Support and protected time for intensive, supervised research career development experience • Biomedical, behavioral, translational research
K12 Mentored Clinical Scientist Program Development Awards	• Support to institutions for the development of independent clinical scientists
K18 Short-term Career Development Award in the Environment Sciences for Established Investigators	• Allow established, well-funded clinician investigators to expand research programs • Answer questions relevant to the environment health sciences • Expand efforts to translational research

(continued)

Name	Description
K22 Career Transition Award	• Support to a post-doctoral fellow in transition to a faculty position
K23 Mentored Patient-Oriented Research Career Development Award	• Support career development • Investigators who have committed to patient-oriented research
K24 Midcareer Investigator Award in Patient-Oriented Research	• Support for clinician investigators to allow protected time for patient-oriented research • Time to act as research mentors
K25 Mentored Quantitative Research Development Award	• To attract quantitative science and engineering investigators who have not previously focused on health and disease-related research
K26 Midcareer Investigator Award in Mouse Pathobiology Research	• Support established pathobiologists • Allow protected time for mouse pathobiology research • Time for mentoring beginning investigators
K30 Clinical Research Curriculum Development	• Attract talented individuals to clinical research • Provide with the skills to translate basic discoveries into clinical treatments

Appendix 3c: National Institutes of Health (NIH) - F, P, and T Series

Type	Name	Description
Individual Fellowship Funding Opportunities (F Series)	F30 F31 Several awards F32 F33	• Assorted fellowships for individuals in MD/PhD and DDS/DMD and PhD programs, for post-doctoral candidates and for senior investigators who wish to make changes in the direction of their research career • Some have specific topics or areas of study
Program Project/ Center Grants (P Series)	P01 Research Program Project Grant P20 Exploratory Grants P30 Center Core Grants P50 Specialized Center	• Multi-project research projects involving a number of independent investigators • Each project relates to a common theme/goal • Support planning activities for large multi-project grants • Support of shared resources/facilities for research by multiple investigators who provide a multidisciplinary approach to a research problem • Support for research and development from basic to clinical • Spectrum of activities comprises multidisciplinary attack on specific disease or biomedical problem

(continued)

Type	Name	Description
Training Grant Funding Opportunities (T Series)	T32 Several awards	• Pre-doctoral and post-doctoral research training opportunities • Early stage graduate research training in the neurosciences, and in reproductive, perinatal, and pediatric epidemiology
	T34 Several awards	• Research training in developmental biology and/or structural birth defects research • Research training and support grants to increase the number of well-prepared students from diverse backgrounds
	T35 Ruth L. Kirschstein National Research Service Award Short-Term Institutional Research Training Grants	• Develop/enhance research training opportunities for careers in biomedical, behavioral, and clinical research
	T36 Minority Access to Research Careers Ancillary Training Activities	• To provide support to under-represented groups to attended training activities to develop knowledge and skills for the pursuit of biomedical research careers
	T90 Training for New Interdisciplinary Research Workforce	• Support for undergraduate, pre-doctoral and post-doctoral students to receive the necessary research experiences to solve complex biomedical and health problems

Appendix 3d: National Institutes of Health (NIH) – Trans-NIH Programs

Name	Description
BECON	• NIH bioengineering consortium
BISTI	• Biomedical Information Science and Technology Initiative
Blueprint	• NIH blueprint for neuroscience research
Diversity Supplements	• Research supplements to promote diversity in health-related research
GWAS	• Genome-Wide Association Studies
PECASE	• Presidential Early Career Award for Scientists and Engineers
Roadmap	• NIH Director's Pioneer Award
	• NIH Director's New Innovator Program

Please note that the information in Appendix 3 pertains to the 2009 funding opportunities. The specific details and availability of funding programs varies from year to year. For current information, please see the NIH website.

Resources

1. National Institutes of Health. About Grants. http://grants.nih.gov/grants/oer.htm. Accessed April 7, 2009.

Appendix 4: Grants at the Canadian Institutes of Health Research (CIHR)

Name	Description
Catalyst Grant	• Short-term to support health research which will lead to more comprehensive opportunities • Pilot or feasibility studies, new tools and methods, etc. • One–three years; up to $100,000/year
Chair	• Policy and program intervention research of national relevance to public health • Support development of graduate and continuing education public health programs • Stimulate innovative approaches to intervention research, mentorship, education, and knowledge translation
Clinician-scientist Salary Award	• Phase 1: stipend for up to six years of training support • Phase 2: salary contribution for up to six years • Up to six years; up to $100,000/year
Doctoral Research Award	• Various fields and amounts available
Emerging Team Grant	• Support new and emerging teams producing high-quality research and providing superior training opportunities • Up to five years; up to $500,000/year
Fellowship	• Various types and amounts available
Knowledge Synthesis Grant/ Synthesis Grant	• To support scoping reviews and syntheses that respond to the information needs of decision makers/knowledge users in all areas of health • To support the use of evidence derived from syntheses by decision makers/knowledge users • Synthesis: up to one year; up to $100,000 • Scoping review: up to one year; up to $50,000
Master's Award	• Recognition and support to students pursuing a Master's degree in a health-related field • Exceptionally high potential for future research achievement is expected • Up to one year; up to $17,500 • Non-renewable
Meetings, Planning, and Dissemination Grant	• Support for meetings to share information, for knowledge exchange and knowledge translation activities • Up to $10,000 for workshops, conferences, etc. On rare occasions up to $25,000. • Non-renewable
Mid-career Investigator Salary Award	• Provide protected time for researchers • Support career re-orientation of researchers to promote entry into high priority areas

(continued)

Name	Description
New Investigator Salary Award	• To provide new investigators with the opportunity to develop and demonstrate their research independence • Up to five years; up to $60,000/year • Non-renewable
Operating Grant	• Support research proposals in all areas of health • No specific requirements for team size, composition, maximum or minimum funds • Usually two–five years • No restrictions on research area, except that randomized controlled trials are not funded
Partnerships for Health System Improvement	• Collaboration between decision makers and researchers to address health system challenges • Any applied health services or policy research topic is applicable
Prize	• Various areas and mandates • Usually recipients must be nominated by a member of the Canadian health research community
Proof of Principle	• To facilitate and improve the commercial transfer of knowledge and technology resulting from academic health research for the benefit of Canadians. • Phase I: up to $150,000/application • Phase II: up to $250,000/application
Randomized Controlled Trials	• Applications for RCTs will be examined for the relevance of the question, appropriateness of methodology, of gender representation, and of subject selection • Applications for dose-finding, safety and efficacy, and non-randomized clinical studies should be made through the operating grant program
Senior Investigator Salary Award	• Support for established investigators • Must be able to devote 75% of time to research
Team Grant	• Support expert teams of talented and experienced researchers • Support the production and translation of new knowledge • Research addressing an important health and disease, health care, or health system problem which is best approached through a collaborative team
Training Grant	• Support the training of researchers that fosters hands-on teamwork within a structured learning environment • Up to $165,000 in first year, after which, up to $325,000/year for maximum of six years
Undergraduate	• Provision of support early in the career • Allow for research experience to encourage subsequent research involvement

Please note that this information pertains to the 2009 funding opportunities. The specific details and availability of funding programs varies from year to year. For current information, please see the CIHR website.

Resources

1. Canadian Institutes of Health Research. 2008–2009 CIHR Grants and Awards Guide. http://www.cihr-irsc.gc.ca/e/22631.html#2-B4. Accessed April 1, 2009.

Appendix 5: Selected Terms Used by the National Institutes of Health (NIH)

Funding Opportunity Announcements (FOA)

NIH Definition: A publicly available document by which a Federal Agency makes known its intentions to award discretionary grants or cooperative agreements, usually as a result of competition for funds. Funding opportunity announcements may be known as program announcements, requests for applications, notices of funding availability, solicitations, or other names depending on the Agency and type of program. Funding opportunity announcements can be found at Grants.gov/FIND and in the NIH Guide for Grants and Contracts.

Targeted Research

NIH Definition: Research funded as a result of an Institute set aside of dollars for a specific scientific area. Institutes solicit applications using research initiatives (RFAs for grants, RFPs for contracts). Targeted research applications are reviewed by chartered peer review committees within Institutes. The opposite is Investigator-Initiated Research.

Initiative

NIH Definition: A request for applications (RFA), request for proposals (RFP), or program announcement (PA) stating the Institute or Center's interest in receiving research applications in a given area because of a programmatic need or scientific opportunity. RFAs and RFPs generally have monies set aside to fund the applications responding to them; program announcements generally do not.

Requests for Applications (RFA)

NIH Definition: The official statement inviting grant or cooperative agreement applications to accomplish a specific program purpose. RFAs indicate the amount of funds set aside for the competition and generally identify a single application receipt date.

Program Announcements (PAs)

NIH Definition: An announcement by an NIH Institute or Center requesting applications in the stated scientific areas. Program Announcements (PA) are published in the NIH Guide for Grants and Contracts.

Request for Proposals (RFP)

NIH Definition: Announces that NIH would like to award a contract to meet a specific need, such as the development of an animal model. RFPs have a single application receipt date and are published in the NIH Guide for Grants and Contracts.

1. National Institutes of Health. Glossary and Acronym List. http://grants.nih. gov/grants/glossary.htm#R. Accessed April 5, 2010.

Subject Index

Note: Appendix page numbers are given with the word "App" after the locators.